Magnetoencephalography

Editors

ROLAND R. LEE
MINGXIONG HUANG

NEUROIMAGING CLINICS OF NORTH AMERICA

www.neuroimaging.theclinics.com

Consulting Editor
SURESH K. MUKHERJI

May 2020 • Volume 30 • Number 2

ELSEVIER

1600 John F. Kennedy Boulevard ● Suite 1800 ● Philadelphia, Pennsylvania, 19103-2899

http://www.neuroimaging.theclinics.com

NEUROIMAGING CLINICS OF NORTH AMERICA Volume 30, Number 2
May 2020 ISSN 1052-5149, ISBN 13: 978-0-323-70940-8

Editor: John Vassallo (j.vassallo@elsevier.com)
Developmental Editor: Casey Potter

Neuroimaging Clinics of North America (ISSN 1052-5149) is published quarterly by Elsevier Inc., 360 Park Avenue South, New York, NY 10010-1710. Months of issue are February, May, August, and November. Business and editorial offices: 1600 John F. Kennedy Blvd., Suite 1800, Philadelphia, PA 19103-2899. Business and editorial offices: 6277 Sea Harbor Drive, Orlando, FL 32887-4800. Periodicals postage paid at New York, NY, and additional mailing offices. Subscription prices are USD 397 per year for US individuals, USD 686 per year for US institutions, USD 100 per year for US students and residents, USD 451 per year for Canadian individuals, USD 874 per year for Canadian institutions, USD 541 per year for international individuals, USD 874 per year for international institutions, USD 100 per year for Canadian students and residents and USD 260 per year for foreign students and residents. To receive student/resident rate, orders must be accompanied by name of affiliated institution, date of term, and the *signature* of program/residency coordinator on institution letterhead. Orders will be billed at individual rate until proof of status is received. Foreign air speed delivery is included in all *Clinics* subscription prices. All prices are subject to change without notice. POSTMASTER: Send address changes to *Neuroimaging Clinics of North America*, Elsevier Health Sciences Division, Subscription **Customer Service, 3251 Riverport Lane, Maryland Heights, MO 63043. Telephone: 1-800-654-2452 (U.S. and Canada); 314-447-8871 (outside U.S. and Canada). Fax: 314-447-8029. E-mail: journalscustomerservice-usa@elsevier.com (for print support); journalsonlinesupport-usa@elsevier.com (for online support).**

Reprints. For copies of 100 or more of articles in this publication, please contact the Commercial Reprints Department, Elsevier Inc., 360 Park Avenue South, New York, NY 10010-1710. Tel.: 212-633-3874; Fax: 212-633-3820; E-mail: reprints@elsevier.com.

Neuroimaging Clinics of North America is covered by *Excerpta Medical/EMBASE,* the RSNA Index of Imaging Literature, *MEDLINE/PubMed (Index Medicus),* MEDLINE/MEDLARS, SciSearch, Research Alert, and Neuroscience Citation Index.

PROGRAM OBJECTIVE

The goal of *Neuroimaging Clinics of North America* is to keep practicing radiologists and radiology residents up to date with current clinical practice in radiology by providing timely articles reviewing the state of the art in patient care.

TARGET AUDIENCE

Practicing radiologists, radiology residents, and other healthcare professionals who utilize neuroimaging findings to provide patient care.

LEARNING OBJECTIVES

Upon completion of this activity, participants will be able to:
1. Review MEG applications for patients with concussions and PTSD; autism, schizophrenia, Alzheimer's disease.
2. Discuss MEG signal processing and techniques for calculating the neuronal sources from measured magnetic signals.
3. Recognize the integration of MEG data with other anatomical and functional brain imaging data-sets.

ACCREDITATION

The Elsevier Office of Continuing Medical Education (EOCME) is accredited by the Accreditation Council for Continuing Medical Education (ACCME) to provide continuing medical education for physicians.

The EOCME designates this journal-based CME activity for a maximum of 10 *AMA PRA Category 1 Credit*(s)™. Physicians should claim only the credit commensurate with the extent of their participation in the activity.

All other healthcare professionals requesting continuing education credit for this enduring material will be issued a certificate of participation.

DISCLOSURE OF CONFLICTS OF INTEREST

The EOCME assesses conflict of interest with its instructors, faculty, planners, and other individuals who are in a position to control the content of CME activities. All relevant conflicts of interest that are identified are thoroughly vetted by EOCME for fair balance, scientific objectivity, and patient care recommendations. EOCME is committed to providing its learners with CME activities that promote improvements or quality in healthcare and not a specific proprietary business or a commercial interest.

The planning committee, staff, authors and editors listed below have identified no financial relationships or relationships to products or devices they or their spouse/life partner have with commercial interest related to the content of this CME activity:
M. Florencia Assaneo, PhD; Susan M. Bowyer, PhD; Richard C. Burgess, MD, PhD; Yu-Han Chen, PhD; Joon Yul Choi, PhD; Suzanne Dikker, PhD; J. Christopher Edgar, PhD; Alberto Fernández, PhD; Heather L. Green, PhD; Anika Guha, MA; Laura Gwilliams, MSc; Matti Hämäläinen, MS; Mingxiong Huang, PhD; Marilu Kelly, MSN, RN, CNE, CHCP; Anne Kösem, PhD; Pradeep Kuttysankaran; Roland R. Lee, MD; Jeffrey David Lewine, PhD; Fernando Maestú, PhD; Junko Matsuzaki, PhD; Gregory A. Miller, PhD; Suresh K. Mukherji, MD, MBA, FACR; Elizabeth W. Pang, PhD; Christos Papadelis, PhD; Andrew C. Papanicolaou, PhD; John Vassallo; Lin Wang, PhD; Zhong Irene Wang, PhD.

The planning committee, staff, authors and editors listed below have identified financial relationships or relationships to products or devices they or their spouse/life partner have with commercial interest related to the content of this CME activity:
Timothy P.L. Roberts, PhD: owns stock in Prism Clinical Imaging and Proteus Neurodynamics; consultant/advisor for AveXis, Inc., CTF MEG International Services LP, Ricoh USA, Inc., and Spago Nanomedical AB.

UNAPPROVED/OFF-LABEL USE DISCLOSURE

The EOCME requires CME faculty to disclose to the participants:
1. When products or procedures being discussed are off-label, unlabelled, experimental, and/or investigational (not US Food and Drug Administration [FDA] approved); and
2. Any limitations on the information presented, such as data that are preliminary or that represent ongoing research, interim analyses, and/or unsupported opinions. Faculty may discuss information about pharmaceutical agents that is outside of FDA-approved labelling. This information is intended solely for CME and is not intended to promote off-label use of these medications. If you have any questions, contact the medical affairs department of the manufacturer for the most recent prescribing information.

TO ENROLL

To enroll in the *Neuroimaging Clinics of North America* Continuing Medical Education program, call customer service at 1-800-654-2452 or sign up online at http://www.theclinics.com/home/cme. The CME program is available to subscribers for an additional annual fee of USD 245.00.

METHOD OF PARTICIPATION

In order to claim credit, participants must complete the following:
1. Complete enrolment as indicated above.

2. Read the activity.
3. Complete the CME Test and Evaluation. Participants must achieve a score of 70% on the test. All CME Tests and Evaluations must be completed online.

CME INQUIRIES/SPECIAL NEEDS

For all CME inquiries or special needs, please contact elsevierCME@elsevier.com.

NEUROIMAGING CLINICS OF NORTH AMERICA

THE CLINICS ARE AVAILABLE ONLINE!
Access your subscription at:
www.theclinics.com

Contributors

CONSULTING EDITOR

SURESH K. MUKHERJI, MD, MBA, FACR
Clinical Professor, Marian University, Director
of Head and Neck Radiology, ProScan
Imaging, Regional Medical Director, Envision
Physician Services, Carmel, Indiana, USA

EDITORS

ROLAND R. LEE, MD
Professor and Director of MEG, MRI, and
Neuroradiology, Department of Radiology,
University of California, San Diego, VA San
Diego Healthcare System, San Diego,
California, USA

MINGXIONG HUANG, PhD
Professor and Co-Director of MEG,
Department of Radiology, UCSD Radiology
Imaging Lab, University of California, San
Diego, VA San Diego Healthcare System, San
Diego, California, USA

AUTHORS

M. FLORENCIA ASSANEO, PhD
Postdoctoral Researcher, Department of
Psychology, New York University, New York,
New York, USA

SUSAN M. BOWYER, PhD
Senior Scientist, Department of Neurology,
MEG Lab, Henry Ford Hospital, Assistant
Professor of Neurology, Wayne State
University School of Medicine, Detroit,
Michigan, USA; Adjust Professor, Department
of Physics, Oakland University, Rochester,
Michigan, USA

RICHARD C. BURGESS, MD, PhD
Director, Magnetoencephalography
Laboratory, Cleveland Clinic Neurological
Institute, Head, Section of Clinical
Neurophysiology, Cleveland Clinic Epilepsy
Center, Professor, Cleveland Clinic Lerner
College of Medicine, The Cleveland Clinic
Foundation, Cleveland, Ohio, USA

YU-HAN CHEN, PhD
Children's Hospital of Philadelphia, CSH115,
Department of Radiology, Philadelphia,
Pennsylvania, USA

JOON YUL CHOI, PhD
Research Fellow, Epilepsy Center,
Neurological Institute, Cleveland Clinic,
Cleveland, Ohio, USA

SUZANNE DIKKER, PhD
Research Scientist, Department of
Psychology, New York University, New York,
New York, USA

J. CHRISTOPHER EDGAR, PhD
Department of Radiology, Research Division,
Lurie Family Foundations MEG Imaging
Center, The Children's Hospital of Philadelphia,
Department of Radiology, Perelman
School of Medicine, University of
Pennsylvania, Philadelphia, Pennsylvania,
USA

ALBERTO FERNÁNDEZ, PhD
Centro de Tecnología Biomédica, Campus de
Montegancedo de la UPM, Department of
Legal Medicine, Psychiatry and Pathology,
Complutense University of Madrid, Madrid,
Spain

HEATHER L. GREEN, PhD
Department of Radiology, Lurie Family
Foundations MEG Imaging Center, The
Children's Hospital of Philadelphia,
Philadelphia, Pennsylvania, USA

ANIKA GUHA, MA
Department of Psychology, University of
California, Los Angeles, Los Angeles,
California, USA

LAURA GWILLIAMS, MSc
PhD Student, Department of Psychology, New
York University, New York, New York, USA;
New York University Abu Dhabi Research
Institute, New York University Abu Dhabi,
Saadiyat Island, Abu Dhabi, United Arab
Emirates

MATTI HÄMÄLÄINEN, MS
Department of Radiology, Athinoula A.
MartinosCenter, Massachusetts General
Hospital, Charlestown, Massachusetts, USA;
Professor of Radiology, Harvard Medical
School, Boston, Massachusetts, USA

MINGXIONG HUANG, PhD
Professor and Co-Director of MEG,
Department of Radiology, UCSD Radiology
Imaging Lab, University of California, San
Diego, VA San Diego Healthcare System, San
Diego, California, USA

ANNE KÖSEM, PhD
Postdoctoral Researcher, Lyon Neuroscience
Research Center (CRNL), Lyon, France

ROLAND R. LEE, MD
Professor and Director of MEG, MRI, and
Neuroradiology, Department of Radiology,
University of California, San Diego, VA San
Diego Healthcare System, San Diego,
California, USA

JEFFREY DAVID LEWINE, PhD
The Mind Research Network, Albuquerque,
New Mexico, USA

FERNANDO MAESTÚ, PhD
Department of Experimental Psychology,
Complutense University of Madrid, Centro de
Tecnología Biomédica, Campus de
Montegancedo de la UPM, Madrid,
Spain

JUNKO MATSUZAKI, PhD
Department of Radiology, Lurie Family
Foundations MEG Imaging Center, The
Children's Hospital of Philadelphia,
Philadelphia, Pennsylvania, USA

GREGORY A. MILLER, PhD
Departments of Psychology, and Psychiatry
and Biobehavioral Sciences, University of
California, Los Angeles, Los Angeles,
California, USA

ELIZABETH W. PANG, PhD
Division of Neurology, The Hospital for Sick
Children, University of Toronto, Toronto,
Ontario, Canada

CHRISTOS PAPADELIS, PhD
Director of Research, Jane and John Justin
Neuroscience Center, Cook Children's Health
Care System, Department of Pediatrics, TCU
and UNTHSC School of Medicine, Fort Worth,
Texas, USA; Laboratory of Children's Brain
Dynamics, Division of Newborn Medicine,
Boston Children's Hospital, Harvard Medical
School, Boston, Massachusetts, USA

ANDREW C. PAPANICOLAOU, PhD
Professor of Neuroscience Emeritus, The
University of Tennessee, College of Medicine,
Memphis, Tennessee, USA

TIMOTHY P.L. ROBERTS, PhD
Department of Radiology, Lurie Family
Foundations MEG Imaging Center, The
Children's Hospital of Philadelphia,
Department of Radiology, Perelman School of
Medicine, University of Pennsylvania,
Philadelphia, Pennsylvania, USA

LIN WANG, PhD
Postdoctoral Researcher, Department of
Psychiatry, Athinoula A. Martinos Center for
Biomedical Imaging, Massachusetts General
Hospital, Harvard Medical School,
Charlestown, Massachusetts, USA

ZHONG IRENE WANG, PhD
Staff Scientist, Epilepsy Center, Neurological
Institute, Cleveland Clinic, Joint Staff,
Department of Biomedical Engineering,
Cleveland Clinic Lerner Research Institute,
Assistant Professor of Medicine, Cleveland
Clinic Lerner College of Medicine of Case
Western Reserve University, Cleveland, Ohio,
USA

Contents

> Magnetoencephalography (MEG) is a noninvasive functional imaging technique for
> the brain. MEG directly measures the magnetic signal due to neuronal activation
> in gray matter with high spatial localization accuracy. The first part of this article
> covers the overall concepts of MEG and the forward and inverse modeling tech-
> niques. It is followed by examples of analyzing evoked and resting-state MEG sig-
> nals using a high-resolution MEG source imaging technique. Next, different
> techniques for connectivity and network analysis are reviewed with examples
> showing connectivity estimates from resting-state and epileptic activity.

> Magnetoencephalography is the noninvasive measurement of miniscule magnetic
> fields produced by brain electrical currents, and is used most fruitfully to evaluate
> epilepsy patients. While other modalities infer brain function indirectly by measuring
> changes in blood flow, metabolism, and oxygenation, magnetoencephalography
> measures neuronal and synaptic function directly with submillisecond temporal res-
> olution. The brain's magnetic field is recorded by neuromagnetometers surrounding
> the head in a helmet-shaped sensor array. Because magnetic signals are not dis-
> torted by anatomy, magnetoencephalography allows for a more accurate measure-
> ment and localization of brain activities than electroencephalography.
> Magnetoencephalography has become an indispensable part of the armamentarium
> at epilepsy centers.

> Noninvasive functional brain imaging with magnetoencephalography (MEG) is regu-
> larly used to map the eloquent cortex associated with somatosensory, motor, audi-
> tory, visual, and language processing before a surgical resection to determine if the
> functional areas have been reorganized. Most tasks can also be performed in the pe-
> diatric population. To acquire an optimal MEG study for any of these modalities, the
> patient needs to be well rested and attending to the stimulation.

Mild traumatic brain injury (mTBI) and posttraumatic stress disorder (PTSD) are leading causes of sustained physical, cognitive, emotional, and behavioral deficits in the general population, active-duty military personnel, and veterans. However, the underlying pathophysiology of mTBI/PTSD and the mechanisms that support functional recovery for some, but not all individuals is not fully understood. Conventional MR imaging and computed tomography are generally negative in mTBI and PTSD, so there is interest in the development of alternative evaluative strategies. Of particular note are magnetoencephalography (MEG) -based methods, with mounting evidence that MEG can provide sensitive biomarkers for abnormalities in mTBI and PTSD.

Magnetoencephalography (MEG) research indicates differences in neural brain measures in children with autism spectrum disorder (ASD) compared to typically developing (TD) children. As reviewed here, resting-state MEG exams are of interest as well as MEG paradigms that assess neural function across domains (e.g., auditory, resting state). To date, MEG research has primarily focused on group-level differences. Research is needed to explore whether MEG measures can predict, at the individual level, ASD diagnosis, prognosis (future severity), and response to therapy.

Schizophrenia (Sz) is a chronic mental disorder characterized by disturbances in thought (such as delusions and confused thinking), perception (hearing voices), and behavior (lack of motivation). The lifetime prevalence of Sz is between 0.3% and 0.7%, with late adolescence and early adulthood, the peak period for the onset of psychotic symptoms. Causal factors in Sz include environmental and genetic factors and especially their interaction. About 50% of individuals with a diagnosis of Sz have lifelong impairment.

As synaptic dysfunction is an early manifestation of Alzheimer disease (AD) pathology, magnetoencephalography (MEG) is capable of detecting disruptions by assessing the synchronized oscillatory activity of thousands of neurons that rely on the integrity of neural connections. MEG findings include slowness of the oscillatory activity, accompanied by a reduction of the alpha band power, and dysfunction of the functional networks. These findings are associated with the neuropathology of the disease and cognitive impairment. These neurophysiological biomarkers predict which patients with mild cognitive impairment will develop dementia. MEG has demonstrated its utility as a noninvasive biomarker for early detection of AD.

This article provides an overview of research that uses magnetoencephalography to understand the brain basis of human language. The cognitive processes and brain networks that have been implicated in written and spoken language comprehension and production are discussed in relation to different methodologies: we review event-related brain responses, research on the coupling of neural oscillations to speech, oscillatory coupling between brain regions (eg, auditory-motor coupling), and neural decoding approaches in naturalistic language comprehension.

Magnetoencephalography (MEG) is a noninvasive neuroimaging technique that measures the electromagnetic fields generated by the human brain. This article highlights the benefits that pediatric MEG has to offer to clinical practice and pediatric research, particularly for infants and young children; reviews the existing literature on adult MEG systems for pediatric use; briefly describes the few pediatric MEG systems currently extant; and draws attention to future directions of research, with focus on the clinical use of MEG for patients with drug-resistant epilepsy.

Multimodal image integration is the procedure that puts together imaging data from multiple sources into the same space by a computerized registration process. This procedure is relevant to patients with difficult-to-localize epilepsy undergoing presurgical evaluation, who typically have many tests performed, including MR imaging, PET, ictal single-photon emission computed tomography, magnetoencephalography (MEG), and intracranial electroencephalogram (EEG). This article describes the methodology of such integration, focusing on integration of MEG. Also discussed is the clinical value of integration of MEG, in terms of planning of intracranial EEG implantation, interpretation of intracranial EEG data, planning of final resection, and addressing surgical failures.

Foreword

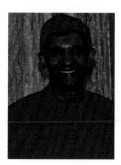

Suresh K. Mukherji, MD, MBA, FACR
Consulting Editor

Magnetoencephalography (MEG) is a powerful functional imaging technique that measures changes in the magnetic fields due to real-time neuronal function. MEG has the ability to reconstruct the neuronal sources of brain activity with spatial resolution of a few millimeters at the cortical level. The first single-channel MEG was measured in 1972, and whole-head MEG units became commercially available in the mid-1990s. There are currently about 20 clinical MEG centers in the United States. So, the $64 million (literally!) question has always been why has such a powerful imaging technique not been widely accepted?

This issue of *Neuroimaging Clinics* focuses on MEG and will help neuroscientists and neuroimagers (like myself!) better understand the "black box." This issue beautifully reviews technique and superbly emphasizes the multiple current clinical applications. I am very grateful to this talented group of article authors for their outstanding contributions. The content and figures are superb, and I want to personally thank each author for their incredible effort.

I would like thank Drs Mingxiong Huang and Roland Lee for editing this superb issue. I especially want to take this opportunity to thank Dr Lee. Roland and I were residents together in the "last century" at the Brigham and Women's Hospital. Roland was (and still is) one of the smartest, talented, and energetic (!) individuals I have ever met. He was always willing to help a junior resident in distress (me), and I feel so privileged to call him a colleague and friend. Thank you to both Roland and your team for this wonderful contribution!

Suresh K. Mukherji, MD, MBA, FACR
Clinical Professor, Marian University
Director of Head & Neck Radiology
ProScan Imaging, Regional Medical Director
Envision Physician Services
Carmel, Indiana, USA

E-mail address:
sureshmukherji@hotmail.com

neuroimaging.theclinics.com

Preface
Magnetoencephalography: Elucidating Brain Function

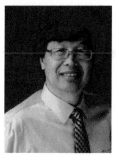   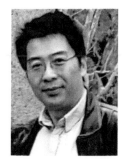

Roland R. Lee, MD   Mingxiong Huang, PhD

Editors

Magnetoencephalography (MEG) is a functional imaging technique that measures the magnetic fields emitted by the brain with millisecond temporal resolution, from which one can reconstruct the neuronal sources of brain activity with spatial resolution of a few millimeters at the cortical level. It differs from most neuroimaging techniques, which generally display a snapshot of brain anatomy; MEG solely elucidates real-time ongoing brain function: neuronal activity. Functional MR imaging is an extremely valuable imaging technique that uses cerebral blood flow as a surrogate for neuronal activity with 3- to 5-second temporal resolution; MEG dispenses with the surrogate blood flow and just measures the brain's neuronal magnetic activity directly, with millisecond temporal resolution!

Although the first single-channel magnetoencephalogram was measured in 1972, and whole-head MEG units became commercially available in the mid-1990s, there are only about 20 clinical MEG centers in the United States. Hence, many readers may not be familiar with MEG, despite the fact that it is formally recognized to be clinically valuable in localization of epileptiform spike activity, and in presurgical mapping of eloquent cortex, and is widely financially reimbursed by federal and private medical insurance.

This issue provides an in-depth exposition of MEG, starting with MEG signal processing, and techniques for calculating the neuronal sources from the measured magnetic signals; then covers the current clinically reimbursed applications of epilepsy and presurgical mapping; then the clinically important topics of MEG used in patients with concussions and posttraumatic stress disorder; and autism. Next are articles on MEG and schizophrenia, Alzheimer disease, and the study of language. We conclude with articles on pediatric MEG, and the integration of MEG data with other anatomical and functional brain imaging data sets.

We are fortunate to have recruited leading national and international expert neuroscientists in MEG to author the articles in this issue, so that the information is thoroughly covered and completely current. After reading this issue, readers will have a complete understanding of MEG's clinical utility as well as its unique role in elucidating brain function.

We thank our friend and colleague, Dr Suresh Mukherji, for inviting us to guest-edit this issue of *Neuroimaging Clinics*. Special thanks for the guidance and patience of John Vassallo, Nick Henderson, and Pradeep Kuttysankaran of Elsevier, who guided us throughout the process.

We dedicate this issue to the memory of two peerless neuroradiologists who recently passed away within a month of each other in late 2017: William G. Bradley, who inspirationally supported and energetically expedited the establishment of our University of California, San Diego MEG Center in 2005; and William W. Orrison, a visionary who recruited us in 1997 to lead his young MEG Center at the Albuquerque VA and gave us our start in

Neuroimag Clin N Am 30 (2020) xv–xvi
https://doi.org/10.1016/j.nic.2020.03.001
1052-5149/20/© 2020 Published by Elsevier Inc.

neuroimaging.theclinics.com

MEG. This issue is a tribute to their inspirational support and mentorship.

Roland R. Lee, MD
Department of Radiology
University of California, San Diego
Radiology Service
VA San Diego Healthcare System
UCSD Radiology Imaging Laboratory
3510 Dunhill Street
San Diego, CA 92121, USA

Mingxiong Huang, PhD
Department of Radiology
University of California, San Diego
Radiology Service
VA San Diego Healthcare System
UCSD Radiology Imaging Laboratory
3510 Dunhill Street
San Diego, CA 92121, USA

E-mail addresses:
rrlee@ucsd.edu (R.R. Lee)
mxhuang@ucsd.edu (M. Huang)

Magnetoencephalography Signal Processing, Forward Modeling, Magnetoencephalography Inverse Source Imaging, and Coherence Analysis

Matti Hämäläinen, MS[a,b], Mingxiong Huang, PhD[c],
Susan M. Bowyer, PhD[d,e,f],*

KEYWORDS

- Magnetoencephalography • Neurons • Parametric source models • Distributed current estimates
- Scanning approaches • Fast-VESTAL • Network connectivity measurement

KEY POINTS

- Magnetoencephalography (MEG) is a noninvasive functional imaging technique for the brain.
- MEG directly measures the magnetic signal due to neuronal activation in gray matter with high spatial localization accuracy, in best cases 2 to 4 mm in the cortex, and high temporal resolution (<1 ms), which also translates into excellent frequency specificity at different frequency bands.
- To localize the neuronal sources and obtain their time-courses, the MEG forward and inverse problems need to be solved.
- The first part of this article covers the overall concepts of MEG and the forward and inverse modeling techniques.
- It is followed by examples of analyzing evoked and resting-state MEG signals using a high-resolution MEG source imaging technique.

MAGNETOENCEPHALOGRAPHY SIGNALS AND THEIR SOURCES

Both magnetoencephalography (MEG) and electroencephalography (EEG) are measures of ongoing neuronal activity, and are ultimately generated by the same sources: postsynaptic currents in groups of neurons that have a geometric arrangement favoring currents with a uniform direction across nearby neurons. The most significant such assembly is that of pyramidal cells in the cerebral cortex. The macroscopic source currents generated by these assemblies, often called the *primary currents*,[1,2] create an electric potential distribution, which can be sampled on the scalp using EEG.

[a] Department of Radiology, Athinoula A. Martinos Center, Massachusetts General Hospital, 149 13th Street, Charlestown, MA 02129, USA; [b] Harvard Medical School, Boston, MA, USA; [c] Department of Radiology, UCSD Radiology Imaging Lab, University of California, San Diego, 3510 Dunhill Street, San Diego, CA 92121, USA; [d] Department of Neurology, MEG Lab, Henry Ford Hospital, 2799 West Grand Boulevard, CFP 079, Detroit, MI 48202, USA; [e] Wayne State University School of Medicine, Detroit, MI, USA; [f] Department of Physics, Oakland University, Rochester, MI, USA
* Corresponding author. Henry Ford Hospital, MEG Lab, 2799 West Grand Boulevard, CFP 079, Detroit, MI 48202.
E-mail address: SBOWYER1@hfhs.org

Neuroimag Clin N Am 30 (2020) 125–143
https://doi.org/10.1016/j.nic.2020.02.001

This potential distribution is associated with passive *volume currents* in the conducting medium.[2] In general, the primary and volume currents together generate the magnetic field, measured with MEG. Rather surprisingly, however, the effect of the volume currents on MEG can be often quite easily taken into account. The integral effect of all the currents to the magnetic field can be computed accurately with a relatively undetailed model of electrical conductivity distribution,[3,4] whereas EEG is significantly affected by the conductivity details between the sources and the electrodes.[5] Furthermore, the effect of the real or virtual reference electrode used has to be correctly taken into account. Because MEG and EEG capture electrical activity patterns of neural populations directly, they allow for functional brain activity to be delineated at a very fine temporal scale and may be decomposed into its dominating oscillatory frequency components.

The ability to compute the MEG/EEG patterns generated by known sources, commonly called the solution of the *forward problem*, opens up the possibility to find an estimate of the primary currents given the MEG measurement. However, this *inverse problem* is ill-posed: many different current distributions are capable of explaining the data (nonuniqueness) and the solutions are sensitive to noise in the data (ill-conditioned). Another way to express the nonuniqueness is to state that there are source distributions that are invisible to MEG, EEG, or both. When one wants to go from the MEG recordings at the sensor level to a plausible estimate of its underlying source, one must accept that one has to *always* use simplifying assumptions and approximations. If one understands the qualities of this simplified equivalent source description it is possible to gain useful insights to brain function from it even though the actual complex spatial details cannot be reliably recovered because the measurements are necessarily made far away from the sources.

One can mitigate the nonuniqueness of the inverse problem by imposing anatomically and physiologically meaningful constraints. The noise sensitivity can be reduced by regularization: exact match between the measured data and those predicted by model is thereby partly sacrificed to make the estimates more robust.[1,6] Interestingly, MEG analysis has from the beginning emphasized the need to work in terms of the source estimates, in the *source space*, rather than with the sensor space signals. In contrast, even today, most of the EEG studies rely on traditional sensor space analyses. The source space approach is, in fact, more straightforward with MEG than with EEG because of the availability of a reasonably accurate forward model and because, as will be discussed later, MEG sees a specific subset of the sources in the brain. The source estimation approach has gradually made its way to EEG analyses as well, emphasizing the benefits of understanding the data in terms of brain sources rather than their manifestations on the scalp or outside the head.

In limited instances, the phenomena observed noninvasively in MEG or EEG can also be accessed with invasive recordings in *humans*. In particular, diagnosis of abnormal epileptic signals often requires the use of invasive electrodes either on the surface of the cortex (electrocorticogram) or in the brain with isolated depth electrodes (stereoelectroencephalogram).

An important concept related to noninvasive and invasive measurements is the *detectability* or signal strength, particularly as a function of the distance between the sensors and the active sources. This depends on three factors: (1) the spatial characteristics of the source; (2) temporal synchrony within the source area; and (3) the spatial selectivity of the sensors. It is well known that at the level of even single neurons or small assemblies of neurons the currents may exhibit a "closed" or "open"configuration.[7] In addition, the contribution of action potentials as opposed to postsynaptic currents is minor at a distance because two opposing current dipoles are needed to represent the primary currents corresponding to action potentials.[8] At a macroscopic level, there may be further cancellation effects caused by the macroscopic curvature of the cortex, in which the primary currents are normal to the cortical mantle.[9] In addition to these spatial effects, the strength of the measured signals depends on the length scale on which the activity is synchronous across cells. If this scale is small, measurements made at a distance, effectively averaging the source currents over a larger area or volume, may have a smaller amplitude than the distance dependence determined by the Maxwell's equations governing the physics would alone predict. This characteristic may explain why high-frequency oscillations, for example, in the gamma band, are often more easily seen in intracranial measures than in extracranial MEG/EEG.[10] Finally, the sensor configuration also needs to be taken into account. This is often described as the lead field, which is the sensitivity pattern of the sensor.[11] It is worth pointing out that invasive recordings with macroscopic electrodes are in many ways similar to the surface EEG measurements, except that some of the electrodes are *potentially* located much closer to the sources than any electrode on the scalp. In principle, source estimation methods similar to those used in MEG/EEG[6] can be used to estimate the sources of the invasive recordings pending an accurate forward model.[12,13] In some cases, simultaneous MEG and invasive recordings are also possible and a combined source estimation approach would allow better resolution of the brain activity than possible based on the surface measures alone.

Because of the ambiguity of the electromagnetic inverse problem it is very difficult to determine the actual extent of the activated areas. In this regard, assuming that the sources of MEG will be confined to the cortical mantle can be useful. For example, it might not be possible to explain the observed signals well with a focal source instead of an extended one because the focal source (current dipole) best explaining the data would not be located in the allowed cortical source space. Conversely, if a cortical constraint is not used a best-fitting dipole source located in the gray matter very likely indicates that the true activity has a limited spatial extent. Some investigators[14] have also argued that the current density supported by brain tissue is remarkably constant across species and brain structures: there seems to be a maximum value across the brain structures and species ($q_0 = 1$–2 nAm/mm^2). The empirical values presented in the work by Murakami and Okada[14] closely matched the theoretic values obtained with an independently validated neural network model, indicating that the invariance is not coincidental. This maximum value leads to a lower limit for the source extent. Because the current dipole density q, (average) dipole amplitude Q, and activated area A are related by $q = Q/A$, and $q < q_0$, we have $A > Q/q_0$. For an estimated current-dipole amplitude $Q = 20$ nAm, the corresponding active cortical area should be $A \geq 10$ mm^2. Similar conclusions can be drawn from the EEG source estimates. However, the dependence of EEG on the tissue conductivities, which are not precisely known, makes it difficult to arrive at reliable quantitative estimates of the source strengths based on EEG only.

Magnetoencephalography Source Estimation

As discussed earlier, the ill-posed nature of the inverse problem makes it difficult to prescribe a universally applicable approach to MEG analysis. However, despite the wide variety of source estimation approaches, to be discussed later, they all share some important common characteristics. First, the elementary *source model* in all approaches is a current dipole, which corresponds to a current source-sink pair with a small separation. Second, the measured data are modeled as a sum of a signal and noise:

$$y(t) = s(t) + n(t)$$

where $y(t) = (y_1(t) \ldots y_M(t))^T$ is a column vector of the measured data in M channels, whereas $s(t) = (s_1(t) \ldots s_M(t))^T$ and $n(t) = (n_1(t) \ldots n_M(t))^T$ are the signal and noise vectors, respectively. It is also usually assumed that the signal and noise are uncorrelated, that is, $E\{n^t s\} = 0$, where $E\{\cdot\}$ indicates the expectation value (over time).

Third, because of the linearity of the Maxwell's equations, the signal amplitudes are linearly related to those of N sources $x(t) = (x_1(t) \ldots x_N(t))^T$ by a gain matrix: $s(t) = Gx(t)$. This relationship is not a "model" in the sense that the matrix G incorporates the *biophysics* of the MEG signal generation and is crucial for understanding the spatial characteristics of MEG. The most basic one is that G is dense, that is, every sensor sees every source with a different weight or, equivalently, each sensor sees a combination of all source activities. Because G is an expression of fundamental laws of physics, it is independent of the neuroscience or clinical question being addressed. For example, one can study the relative sensitivities of MEG/EEG to sources at different cortical sites and gain understanding to the relative merits of the two types of measurements with the help of just the solution of the forward problem without a need to specify or apply a source estimation procedure first.[15] In practice, the time is discretely sampled, and the relationship between the data, source amplitudes, and noise can be compactly expressed as $Y = GX + N$, where the columns of the matrices Y, X, and N are the samples of the data, source amplitudes, and noise at times t_k, $k = 1 \ldots K$.

Finally, it is usually assumed that the noise is uncorrelated across time points and that at each time point the noises in different channels are jointly Gaussian with time-independent covariance matrix C_n, which is estimated either from data acquired in the absence of a subject ("empty room data") or from periods of the recording when signals of interest are not present. The former approach is used when sources of spontaneous activity, including epileptic spikes, are to be estimated while the latter approach applies to evoked-response measurements. Once C_n has been estimated, the data y and the gain matrix G are usually whitened to allow for uniform treatment in all source estimation approaches. These whitened quantities are obtained by the transformations $\tilde{y} = C_n^{-1/2} y$ and $\tilde{G} = C_n^{-1/2} G$, where $C_n^{-1/2}$ is the inverse of the square root of C_n. After whitening, $\tilde{n}_k \sim N(0, 1)$ and the whitened noise covariance $\tilde{C}_n = I$, which simplifies the subsequent analysis.

With this background, the task of MEG source estimation is to find best estimates $\hat{\boldsymbol{x}}(t)$ given the measured data $\boldsymbol{y}(t)$, the gain matrix $\boldsymbol{G}$, and characteristics of noise $\boldsymbol{n}(t)$. The following sections discuss the particular approaches used to compute $\boldsymbol{G}$, that is, the forward models, followed by an overview of different source estimation techniques.

Forward models

In order for the MEG source estimation (inverse modeling) task to succeed we need to possess an accurate enough forward model, which consists of a description of the distribution electrical conductivity of the head and an analytical or numerical method to compute MEG (and EEG), given the conductivity assumptions and the elementary sources, the source model. Notably, the magnetic permeability of the head is close enough to that of the vacuum and the time derivatives can be ignored from the Maxwell's equations for the computation of MEG. Therefore, the quasistatic approximation[1,16] is sufficient. This means that the effects of the changes in source amplitudes $\boldsymbol{x}$ on the measured data $\boldsymbol{y}$ are instantaneous: there are no propagation delays or capacitive effects. Thus, if there is a change in the measured spatial MEG distribution, the source distribution or noise has changed. For the following discussion it must be noted that the electrical conductivity is not only a location-dependent scalar quantity but may also possess anisotropy: the conductivity differs depending on the direction in which it is measured. This anisotropy can be measured not only with direct electrical means but also with help of diffusion-weighted MR imaging.[17]

The simplest and a surprisingly good approximation for the head's conductivity distribution for MEG relies on spherical symmetry: the head is assumed to be composed of spherical shells with different electrical conductivities. In this case, a closed-form analytical expression exists for the magnetic field (MEG) outside the sphere.[18–20] This sphere model yields MEG characteristics of remarkable simplicity. First, unlike in EEG, only currents tangential to the surface contribute to the magnetic field. Because the principal direction of the primary currents in the cortex is perpendicular to the cortex, there are important differences between MEG and EEG. Specifically, EEG receives overwhelming contributions from the activity in the gyri, close to the electrodes. This sensitivity to nearby sources may often overshadow the signals from the more distant sulci, which MEG is primarily sensitive to. Furthermore, if the synchronous activity is extended over a large area of cortex covering both walls of a sulcus and the adjacent gyri, the MEG signals from the sulcal walls cancel out, whereas the gyral activity with currents pointing radially in the same direction at the gyri will be still seen in EEG.[9]

Second, the radial component of the magnetic field can be computed directly from the primary current, and even the tangential components can be computed without explicit reference to the volume currents. Third, unlike for EEG, the result is independent of the conductivity profile along the model's radius. Although these assertions are not strictly correct under more realistic conductivity assumptions, they serve as a good baseline with respect to which differences can be often considered as small perturbations. Furthermore, although the analytical approach is by far the most efficient and accurate one for the sphere model, the numerical methods described later can be applied in the spherically symmetric case as well, emphasizing the dichotomy between the model assumptions and the actual solution method used. It should be also noted that other simple conductor shapes, including the ellipsoid, can be handled analytically.[18]

If the spherical symmetry is abandoned and the head is assumed to consist of homogeneous compartments of realistic shape, the solution can be obtained with the boundary-element method (BEM).[3,21] This numerical approach has been finessed and can now even take into account thin layers of CSF.[22] In addition, it has been shown that the BEM can incorporate compartment topologies earlier believed to be only accessible with finite-element method (FEM) and finite-difference method.[23] Specifically, the limitation to nested (layered) and island-in-the-sea geometries can be relaxed. The latter development is particularly important for the infant head: the infant skull consists of separate pieces that are connected by soft tissue (fontanels). In this geometry, each piece of skull shares its single closed boundary surface with the scalp, fontanel, and brain, resulting in piecewise-constant conductivity contrast across this boundary. Previous attempts to model this geometry using BEM have used an approximation in which the fontanel is taken into account with a thinner region in the skull.[24] For the purposes of MEG modeling in adults, it is, however, often sufficient to consider the skull to be a perfect insulator.[3,25] However, it has been later established that a three-compartment model consisting of the intracranial space, skull, and the scalp is preferable even for MEG[26] and certainly if combined analysis of MEG and EEG is contemplated.[27] Routine use of multicompartment models, however, depends on using accurate and reliable MR imaging–based means to estimate the shape of the skull compartment. Furthermore, the determination of the electrical conductivity of each compartment remains a challenge.

The prevailing approach in computing the MEG/EEG forward solutions in complex conductor geometries is the FEM, which has been significantly developed.[28–34] The FEM can incorporate an arbitrary conductivity distribution, including anisotropies. However, especially given the uncertainties in the conductor geometry and the actual electrical conductivities, and possibly the need to resort to atlas-based approximate models, the modern BEM approaches offer several benefits: (1) because the potential is computed on the boundary surfaces only, the intricate methods to accommodate the source singularities in the volume-based FEM are not needed. (2) Thin layers of cerebrospinal fluid (CSF), or touching surfaces can be accommodated by locally increasing the density of the surface tessellations rather than having to create a large number of voxel elements. (3) The computational burden is small enough to allow a detailed study of the effects of the conductivity geometry, conductivities, and surface tessellation density on the accuracy of the solution. On the other hand, the FEM offers the capability to model anisotropic conductivity, possibly important in the white matter[35] and the skull.[36]

The refinement of the forward model increases the precision of the source locations estimated (reduces bias). However, in general, an improved forward model does not increase the spatial resolution, if understood as the ability to resolve nearby simultaneously active sources. In some cases, the source estimates may actually be relatively insensitive to the accuracy of the forward model.[37]

Overview of source estimation approaches
The aim of the solution of the inverse problem is to produce source estimates, which correctly describe the locations and extents of the sources underlying the measured MEG data, and yield the unmixed waveforms of the underlying sources. The MEG/EEG source estimation methods can be divided into 3 categories: (1) parametric source models, (2) distributed current estimates, and (3) scanning approaches.

In the parametric approach one assumes that the cortical activity underlying the measurements is sparse, that is, salient activity occurs only in a small number of cortical sites, and that each active area has a small enough spatial extent to be equivalently accounted for by a point source, a current dipole. These single or multidipole models have been very successful in the analysis of

evoked potentials and fields.[38–40] Even though the multidipole model is often used to explain measurements of primary and secondary sensory responses, it has also been employed in modeling of more complex cognitive functions, see, for example Refs.[41,42], and cortical rhythms.[43] The current dipole model is the current clinical standard in the analysis of MEG data for the established clinical applications of MEG: localization of epileptic spikes and mapping of eloquent cortex before surgery. In addition to considering the estimated dipole amplitudes and the locations when evaluating the validity of the dipole model, rigorous statistical criteria have been applied as well. Once the model parameters have been estimated, the significance of the model can be evaluated by using a χ^2 statistic. If one cannot reject the dipole model, the confidence region can be computed to verify that the model parameters are significant, that is, that the model is identifiable. These basic straightforward statistical criteria are still rather rarely systematically applied even though they were introduced to MEG analytical tools more than 25 years ago.[20]

The distributed modeling approaches assume a distribution of sources on the cortex and other structures and apply an additional criterion to select a particular distribution that explains the data and produces an image of the most likely current distribution. Most, if not all, of these methods can be expressed either by using the Bayesian statistical framework or by expressing the best estimate, $\widehat{x}$, as a solution of the optimization problem:

$$\widehat{x} = \underset{x}{\operatorname{argmin}}\left\{ \tilde{y} - \tilde{G}x_2^2 + f(x)\right\}$$

where the first data term promotes agreement of the actual data and those predicted by the model according to the ℓ_2-norm criterion, and $f(x)$ is the additional criterion (in Bayesian terms, related to the prior) for the source amplitudes x.

To date, the most widely used approach of this kind is the cortically constrained minimum-norm estimate (MNE),[44–46] which constrains the currents to the cortical mantle and selects a solution, which has the minimum overall power, that is, $f(x) = \lambda^2 x^T x$, where λ^2 is a positive regularization constant. The MNE is a diffuse estimate, usually overestimating the extent of the source, and therefore, the extent of the MNE should not be interpreted literally. In addition to the ℓ_2-norm constraint used in MNE, it is possible to use a criterion promoting sparsity, for example, the ℓ_1-norm to produce minimum-current estimates (MCEs), which resemble multiple dipole models with the difference that the constellation of sources is different at each time point.[47] Subsequent developments of ℓ_1-norm solutions (mixed-norm estimates) have included constraints on the source waveforms and the requirement that the set of sources remains unchanged throughout the analysis period.[48–50] Starting from a slightly different viewpoint, related source estimation methods promoting sparse solutions have also been introduced. These include magnetic field tomography,[51] Multi-Resolution FoCal Underdetermined System Solution (MR-FOCUSS),[52] and VEctor-based Spatial-Temporal Analysis on an L1-minimum-norm solution (VESTAL).[53,54] The Fast-VESTAL approach[54] is discussed later in more detail.

One way to characterize the different distributed estimation approaches is to use time-space plots shown in **Fig.1**. As shown, every source location in the standard MNE (ℓ_2) has a nonzero time-course (see **Fig. 1A**). This means that if the SNR could be increased indefinitely, every location becomes significantly active, albeit with different amplitudes. Because this estimate is linear in the data, the time-courses of the sources are linear combinations of the sensor time-courses and thus have same general time-frequency structure.

In the MCE (ℓ_1) case, the solution is nonlinear in the data, and each time point is considered separately. Therefore, the constellation of sources changes as a function of time and the time-course at a given source location has a nonphysiologic telegraphic characteristic (see **Fig. 1B**). When applied MCE to actual source analysis, several nearby source sites are usually averaged together to yield more believable source waveforms. To avoid this heuristic procedure in favor of a more principled approach, the authors introduced the mixed ℓ_{21}-norm estimate.[48–50] In this method, the source waveforms are assumed to be weighted sums of (orthonormal) temporal functions. The selection of the temporal waveform series coefficients, different for each source location, is based on the ℓ_2 norm, whereas the ℓ_1 norm is used over space (see **Fig. 1C**). This method results

in a sparse constellation of sources, which is constant over time. The authors used the SVD of the data matrix $Y = USV^T$ to yield the series of temporal component waveforms as a subset of columns of V. This particular ℓ_{21}-norm estimate (MxNE) thus has the temporal characteristics of the original data, similar to the ℓ_2-norm MNE. As a result, each of the sources will be active throughout the analysis period.

To comply with a scenario where the source constellation may change over the analysis period, the authors introduced the time-frequency mixed-norm estimate (**Fig. 1D**). This method uses a combination of ℓ_{21} and ℓ_1 norms over the time-frequency coefficients of the data[49]. Without going to details, the method promotes source waveforms that are locally smooth but globally sparse. In other words, the sources may turn on and off, and the source constellation is thus allowed to change over time.

In the third approach to source estimation, a suitable scanning function, derived from the input data, is evaluated at each candidate source location. A high value indicates a likely location of a source. Examples of this method are the linearly constrained minimum variance beamformer[55,56] and multiple signal classification (MUSIC)[39,40] approaches. The beamformer method has gained a lot of popularity among MEG researchers, whereas its use in EEG has been limited. This is probably due to the fact that for the beamformer method to work, the forward model needs to be sufficiently accurate.[57] Finally, the scanning approaches differ from the parametric dipole model and the source imaging approaches in the sense that the "pseudoimages" they produce do not constitute a current distribution that is capable of directly explaining the measured data.

All three types of methods have been widely used for the analysis of cortical activity and have also been validated to varying degrees in patients with invasive recordings, see, for example, Ref.[58] However, subcortical structures and the cerebellum also play important roles in brain function.

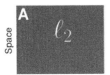
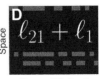
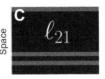

Fig. 1. Sparsity patterns promoted by the different distributed source estimates: (A) ℓ_2 all non-zero, (B) ℓ_1 scattered and unstructured non-zero, (C) ℓ_{21} block row structure, and (D) $\ell_{21} + \ell_1$ block row structure with intra-row sparsity. Gray color indicates non-zero coefficients. TF Coeff, time-frequency coefficients. (*Adapted from* Gramfort A, Strohmeier D, Haueisen J, et al. Time-frequency mixed-norm estimates: sparse M/EEG imaging with non-stationary source activations. NeuroImage 2013 70:410-422; with permission. https://doi.org/10.1016/j.neuroimage.2012.12.051.)

For example, brainstem and thalamic relay nuclei have a central role in sensory processing.[59,60] Thalamocortical and hippocampal oscillations govern states of sleep, arousal, and anesthesia.[61] Striatal regions are crucial for movement planning, whereas limbic structures such as the hippocampus and amygdala drive memory, emotion, and learning.[62–64] Unfortunately, the anatomy of the brain poses two particular challenges for deep source estimation with MEG. First, deep brain structures are farther away from the sensors than the cerebral cortex and thus produce much lower-amplitude MEG signals than the cortex. A second, perhaps more fundamental, problem stems from the fact that the subcortical structures are surrounded by the cortical mantle. As a result, measurements arising from the activity of deep structures can, in principle, be explained by a surrogate distribution of currents on the cortical surface. This ambiguity also means that it is even harder to estimate subcortical activity when cortical activity is occurring simultaneously.

However, Krishnaswamy and colleagues[65] reasoned that these limitations could be mitigated if only a finite number of cortical sites are active together with the subcortical structures. In many neuroscience studies, salient cortical activity at any moment in time tends to be restricted to a small set of well-circumscribed areas. It follows that if we can identify this sparse subset of active cortical sources and eliminate the remaining irrelevant cortical sources,[66] we have a chance at recovering the locations and time-courses of both cortical and subcortical sources. Krishnaswamy and colleagues[65] also demonstrated the feasibility of this approach by introducing a new source estimation method capitalizing on this insight. Its general applicability will depend on the degree of overlap among the MEG field patterns the source candidates and the signal-to-noise ratio of the measurements.

INTRODUCTION TO SPATIOTEMPORAL L1 MINIMUM-NORM SOLUTIONS

High-resolution MEG inverse imaging methods have been developed to overcome the limitations of dipole fit and beamformer approaches while maintaining high spatial resolutions. VESTAL[53] and Fast-VESTAL[54,67] used temporal information in the data to enhance the stability of the reconstructed L1-minimum norm solution. In addition, not coincidentally, because this approach makes no additional assumptions about the temporal dynamics of the sources, it can also handle sources that are highly correlated.

Using simulations and human MEG data, it was shown that Fast-VESTAL (1) can accurately localize many dipolar and nondipolar sources; (2) can localize and resolve 100% correlated sources, uncorrelated sources, and anything in between; (3) is able to faithfully recover source time-courses; (4) has robustness to different SNR conditions (including SNR with negative dB levels); (5) requires no predetermination of the number of sources (model order); and (6) can provide statistical maps of MEG source images. Here, the authors present examples applying the updated Fast-VESTAL algorithm to obtain high spatial and temporal source images in human evoked and resting-state MEG examinations.

Previous versions of Fast-VESTAL are described in Refs.[54,67] The updated development of Fast-VESTAL adopted a generalized second-order cone programming for the minimum L1-norm solver. One interesting feature of Fast-VESTAL is its optimal depth weighting based on the lead fields. This procedure allows Fast-VESTAL to accurately localize sources in depths. Another valuable feature of Fast-VESTAL is that it can be used directly for analyzing resting-state MEG signal (see later discussion) via an automated selection of dominant modes using the objective prewhitening method.[54]

FAST-VESTAL's APPLICATIONS TO EVOKED MAGNETOENCEPHALOGRAPHY EXAMINATIONS

In this section, the authors provide an example of using Fast-VESTAL to localize evoked MEG responses, in this case the relatively straightforward human MEG median-nerve responses.

Localize Median-Nerve Magnetoencephalographic Responses

Fast-VESTAL was applied to a data set containing MEG responses evoked by left median-nerve stimulation in a healthy subject. **Fig. 2**A shows the measured sensor-waveforms of MEG responses using an Elekta/Neuromag Vector view system evoked by right median-nerve stimulation, with 204 gradiometers. The averaged sensor waveforms from about 300 artifact-free epochs were used in the analysis. The predicted MEG sensor waveforms in **Fig. 2**B from the Fast-VESTAL solution matched the measurement very well. **Fig. 2**C shows that mainly noise remained in the residual waveforms (ie, measured minus predicted). The superimposed source time-courses are plotted in **Fig. 2**D.

The middle panel of **Fig. 2** shows the spatial maps of 2 representative sources obtained by

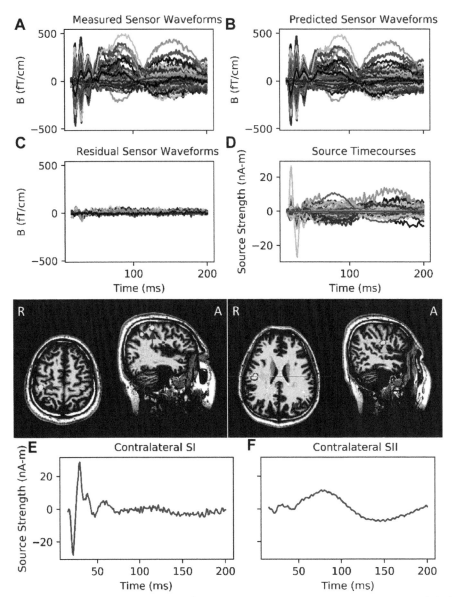

Fig. 2. High-resolution MEG source images of median-nerve responses using Fast-VESTAL. (*A*) shows the measured sensor-waveforms of MEG responses evoked by the right median-nerve stimulation. (*B*) The predicted MEG sensor waveforms from the Fast-VESTAL solution matched the measurement very well. (*C*) Shows that mainly noise remained in the residual waveforms (ie, measured minus predicted). (*D*) The superimposed source time-courses are shown. The middle panels show the spatial maps of two representative sources obtained by Fast-VES-TAL for the responses evoked by the left median nerve stimulation: one in contralateral (right) primary somato-sensory cortex (cSI, red arrows), and another in contralateral secondary somatosensory areas (cSII, green arrows). (*E, F*) The plots of the strength of the current flow over the time-courses for each source.

Fast-VESTAL for the responses evoked by left median nerve stimulation: one in contralateral (right) primary somatosensory cortex (cSI, red arrows) and another in contralateral secondary somatosensory areas (cSII, green arrows). The plots in Fig. 2E and F show the time-courses of the 2 sources from Fast-VESTAL. The cSI time-course showed sharp early components that peaked at ~20 ms and ~30 ms with opposite polarities (Fig. 2E). These early, sharp, and transient components were due to thalamocortical interactions.[68] The time-courses of the cSII source had 2 slow peaks with latencies at ~75 ms and ~140 ms, respectively (see Fig. 2F), mostly due to cortico-cortical interactions.[53,54,69–72] This example illustrates Fast-VESTAL's high-resolution source images with high degree of agreement with known electroneurophysiology.[68]

FAST-VESTAL's APPLICATIONS TO RESTING-STATE MAGNETOENCEPHALOGRAPHY EXAMINATIONS

Resting-state MEG (rs-MEG) has been used to assess abnormalities in neurologic and/or psychiatric disorders such as mild traumatic brain injury[73,74] and posttraumatic stress disorder (PTSD),[75] as well as to study the normal brain functions. This is because of rs-MEG's simplicity in data acquisition and its insensitivity to the performance variability of the testing subjects. In this section, the authors present examples of Fast-VESTAL source images obtained from healthy subjects and examples of applying rs-MEG Fast-VESTAL source imaging in detecting abnormal activity in PTSD neurocircuitry.

Fast-VESTAL Resting-State Magnetoencephalographic Images in Healthy Subjects

Fast-VESTAL was used to obtain the source amplitude (root mean square) images of human resting-state (eyes-closed) MEG signals from 41 healthy control subjects and from 41 sets of empty-room data.[54] In each human and empty-room data set, the MEG sensor covariance matrix for the resting-state recording was calculated for 4 different frequency bands, namely in alpha (8–12 Hz), beta (15–30 Hz), gamma (30–100 Hz), and low-frequency (1–7 Hz) bands. **Fig. 3** shows the Fast-VESTAL source images (t-score) transformed from the subject's native coordinates to the standard MNI-152 atlas coordinates. Resting-state alpha-band activity detected by EEG[76] and MEG[77,78] is known to be strong in the posterior half of the head (occipital, parietal, and posterior temporal regions) but may extend into the central areas in regions that generate the rolandic mu rhythm, see reviews in Refs.[79,80] The results obtained from Fast-VESTAL for the alpha-band were highly consistent with this neurophysiology. **Fig. 3** builds on this knowledge by providing a more refined analysis of the generators of human alpha-band activity. For example, within the occipital lobe, activity from intracalcarine, supracalcarine, and lateral-occipital cortices was clearly distinguishable in the Fast-VESTAL source images (see **Fig. 3**). Likewise, it has not been clear whether the alpha-band activities in the central sulcus area (ie, the rolandic mu rhythm) are mainly from the postcentral gyrus (primary somatosensory cortex), the precentral gyrus (primary motor cortex), or both. The Fast-VESTAL source images in the alpha band showed that although alpha activity extended to the precentral gyrus, the dominant activity was clearly from the postcentral gyrus, more specifically from the hand representation area of the somatosensory cortex.

The Fast-VESTAL source-amplitude images for the generation of the beta-band MEG signals were also highly consistent with previous EEG and MEG findings. Beta-band activities from the pre- and postcentral gyri are part of the rolandic mu rhythm.[80] The Fast-VESTAL source images further showed that the postcentral gyri beta-band

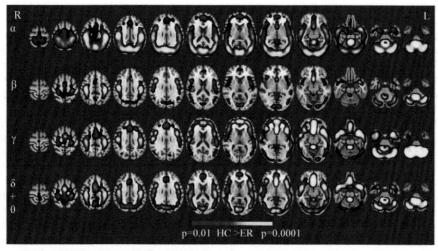

Fig. 3. Whole-brain rs-MEG source-amplitude images averaged from 41 healthy control (HC) subjects against empty room (ER) in MNI-152 atlas coordinates from Fast-VESTAL in alpha (first row), beta (second row), gamma (third row), and low-frequency (delta plus theta, fourth row) bands.

(mu) activity is mainly from the hand representation area of the somatosensory cortex, consistent with previous MEG research.[81]

The gamma-band source amplitude images from Fast-VESTAL also clearly showed larger involvement of frontal generators, different from those previously observed in alpha or beta bands (see **Fig. 3**). Interestingly, gamma-band activity was also found in the anterior hippocampi, the amygdala, and the temporal pole. These results suggest that MEG resting-state gamma-band signal may be useful for studying memory and emotion processing. Fast-VESTAL–based MEG source amplitude images were also derived for low-frequency bands: delta (1–4 Hz) and theta (4–7 Hz) bands. The locations of midline frontal activity in paracingulate gyrus, medial frontal cortices, and subcallosal cortices seem to be consistent with theta activity seen in EEG, even though most of the EEG studies were task activated (eg, problem solving) and provided no specific information on source locations.[80,82–85] Another interesting finding from the Fast-VESTAL result is the high degree of similarity between gamma band and delta-theta band for the inferior frontal and anterior temporal regions (see **Fig. 3**).

This example demonstrates the strengths of obtaining high-resolution rs-MEG images using Fast-VESTAL. This study established the normative database in healthy control subjects, which will be used in assessing abnormalities in neurologic and/or psychiatric disorders.

COHERENCE IMAGING FOR NETWORK ANALYSIS

Communication or connectivity from different regions of the brain occurs along pathways that connect these different areas of the brain.[86] The signals that are sent along these networks (nodes and pathways) arise from the oscillations of the neurons. Synchronized oscillating neurons provide the information flow within the cortex. MEG is a noninvasive way to detect the neuronal oscillations that provide the network of communication across the brain.[87] Detection of the frequency content and time lags of the synchronous oscillating neurons firing can be used as a guide to determine connections in the brain that are sending or receiving information. Brain connectivity networks can be subdivided into 3 main categories: neuroanatomical, functional, and effective connectivity.[88–90] In this section functional connectivity in the frequency domain will be reviewed to show how coherence can be used to look at areas of the brain that are hyperactive and continually communicating with other regions of the brain,

as is the case in patients with epilepsy. Coherence is one mathematical method that can detect how well 2 or more brain regions with similar oscillatory activity are connected with each other. Phase synchrony is another method that can be used to determine if these oscillatory activities are in sync or out of sync with each other. Analysis can be performed on these connectivity results to provide evidence of abnormal network activity in patients, such as epilepsy, schizophrenia, and autism. The detection of local and widespread network interactions may provide greater promise for determining the laterality of epilepsy ictal onset zones and/or for defining the surgical target.[91] In schizophrenia patients or autistic patients they may provide a biomarker to test drug effects. The interest in detecting and understanding the functional properties of the brain's networks is motivating the development of advanced mathematical imaging techniques and analysis. This in turn provides for the need to understand the different techniques for measuring and for analyzing the location and strengths of these functional brain networks.[92,93] For a review of mathematical equations of connectivity measures used in EEG and MEG for neurologic disorders see Ref.[90] or Ref.[89]

Functional Connectivity

Functional connectivity is established by identifying correlations of activity between multiple regions of the brain involved in primary brain function or higher order information processing. During cognitive and sensory processing, brain activity is characterized by bursts of information flow and correlated network activity. These bursts of regional brain activity are called nodes and the links to other nodes are called pathways. These regions (nodes) may only be active for a short period of time, which emphasizes the dynamic fluctuation of information flowing around the brain during cognitive or sensory processing, or they may be active for minutes, hours, or even days as in the case of the epileptic network.[94] Further, brain networks have frequency-dependent characteristics that differ between local or global pathways in the brain. Functional connectivity studies in patients with schizophrenia have shown beta- and gamma-band activities are abnormal.[95] The dysfunctional oscillations in these frequencies may be due to abnormalities in the rhythm generating networks of gamma-aminobutyric acid (GABA) interneurons and corticocortical connections.[96] Coherence and phase synchrony are common mathematical methods for quantifying frequency-dependent coordination of brain activity. Functional connectivity does not determine the specific direction of information flow in the brain or an underlying structural model. It just shows that these regions are connected. Functional connectivity information is contained in brain signals recorded by both EEG and MEG. Results from network analysis provides for the coherent locations to be imaged directly into the specific regions of the brain (called source space); in past years coherence was seen by connecting lines between electrodes or coils that had similar frequency profiles on the brain surface (called sensor space).

Neurons

Connectivity measures of the brain are performed to map out the communication networks needed for the brain to function. These networks are made up of neurons that function in unison to send signals to other parts of the brain. There are several properties of the neuron that play an important role in generating membrane potential oscillations that can be detected by neuroimaging devices. Neurons communicate with other neurons by releasing one of more than 50 different types of neurotransmitters in the brain, some of which are excitatory (stimulate the brain) and some are inhibitory (calm the brain).[97] Voltage-gated ion channels generate action potentials and periodic spiking membrane potentials that produce oscillatory activity and facilitate synchronous activity in neighboring neurons.[98,99] Coherent neuronal communications are based on neurotransmission dynamics dictated by major neurotransmitters such as the amino acids glutamate and GABA. Other important neurotransmitters include acetylcholine, dopamine, adrenaline, histamine, serotonin, and melatonin.[100–102] There is growing evidence that glutamatergic dysregulation may underlie schizophrenia and psychosis.[97]

Synchronized activity of large numbers of neurons can give rise to large magnetic field and electric field oscillations, which are detected by EEG/MEG,[1] and the secondary metabolic responses are detected by functional MR imaging/PET.[103] Coherent activity within the whole brain is evidence for a network of dynamic links (pathways) between different brain regions (nodes) that distribute information.[104] Detection of normal or abnormal networks can provide information on the underlying developmental and/or neurologic disorder.

Effective Connectivity

Effective connectivity is the next processing step that would need to be evaluated to determine in which direction the signals are flowing in the brain.[93,105] Using mathematical techniques such as Granger causality or transfer entropy, locations in the brain can be identified as a sender or receiver of the information flowing in the brain. MEG has been used to show the flow of information in the brain networks during a right finger tapping task using the dynamic imaging of coherent sources method.[106] The functional connectivity for approximately 8 Hz found highly coherent areas in the right cerebellum, left thalamus and left primary motor cortex (M1), and left premotor cortex (PMC). Further analysis quantifying the strength and direction of the motor movement was seen flowing from cerebellum to thalamus, to PMC, to M1, to cerebellum.[106]

Functional and effective connectivity techniques depend on calculating the communication of active neural signals that are oscillating over short and long periods of time. Techniques such as EEG and MEG, with their excellent temporal resolution, are optimal for calculating connectivity.[89,90] MEG and EEG data are usually filtered and have noise artifacts removed before advanced analysis. In many cases it is helpful to first decompose the signal into temporal and spatial modes using techniques such as principal component analysis or independent component analysis (ICA). These techniques can be used to extract noise artifacts, such as cardiac activity, from the data or to identify a particular signal of interest, such as an epileptic seizure before imaging.

NETWORK CONNECTIVITY MEASUREMENT

Network connectivity measurements can be measured in the frequency domain with methods such as coherence and phase synchrony and in the time domain with methods such as correlation and Granger Causality.

Coherence

Coherence is a measure of the synchronicity of the neuronal oscillations. Coherence analysis is a mathematical technique that can be applied to study the functional relationship between spatially separated scalp electrodes (EEG) or coils (MEG) and to estimate the similarities of waveform components generated by the neurons in the underlying cortical regions.[107] The coherence results are used to determine if different areas of the brain are generating signals that are significantly correlated or coherent with each other and would have a number close to 1; or not significantly correlated with each other and would have a number close to 0. Coherence differs from correlation in that the assessment of brain synchrony is done for very narrow frequency bands where the band activity is quantified by an amplitude and phase. These transient waveform oscillations can be quantified by first applying a fast Fourier transform (FFT), which is a time-frequency decomposition technique. This generates a sequence of amplitude/phase components for each narrow frequency bin of the FFT that spans the frequency content of the data. After transformation to a time-frequency representation, the strength of network interactions can be estimated by calculation of coherence, which is a measure of synchrony between signals from different brain regions for each FFT frequency component. This is the most common measure to describe how 2 or more time series are related. Strictly speaking coherence is a statistic that is used to determine the relationship between 2 data sets. It is used to determine if the signal content of 2 inputs are the same or different. If the signals measured by 2 electrodes or coils are identical then they have a coherence value of 1; depending on how dissimilar they are the coherent value will approach 0. It is commonly used to estimate the spectral densities of 2 signals and so is equivalent to a correlation coefficient in the frequency domain. Unlike correlation, coherence has a range of 0 to 1, and because each FFT yields one pair of FFT components, multiple independent segments of data are needed for evaluation.[108]

As mentioned earlier this technique can be applied to the MEG and EEG waveforms in sensor space or it can be applied to the localized MEG solutions in source space. Coherence has been widely used in studying epileptiform activity to determine seizure onset zones. In sensor space Song and colleagues[109] showed that EEG coherence can be used to characterize a pattern of strong coherence centered on temporal lobe structures in several patients with epilepsy. Hinkley and colleagues[95] used source space MEG to detect decreased and increased connectivity differences between patients with schizophrenia and control subjects that may prove to be important target areas for treatment. In source space, Elisevich and colleagues[110] showed that MEG coherence source imaging in the brain can provide targets for successful surgical resections in patients with epilepsy. In this study 10 minutes of rs-MEG data were acquired and band pass filtered 3 to 50 Hz from 30 patients and 11 controls. Data were divided into 80 segments, each containing 7.5 seconds of data,[52,111] each data segment had the signals from neuronal sources isolated using an ICA spatiotemporal decomposition technique designed to extract signals from compact sources that exhibited burst behavior with minimal temporal overlap with other active sources. These ICA signal components have MEG spatial magnetic field patterns corresponding to one or a few spatially distinct compact sources, which are much easier to image accurately using the MR-FOCUSS, a current distribution source imaging technique.[52] Simultaneously a separate algorithm calculated the cross-spectrum between these ICA signals. In these cross-spectrum calculations, a sequence of FFT spectra was calculated using 0.5 second windows and 25% overlap with FFT amplitudes for 24 frequency bins of 2 Hz width between 3 and 50 Hz. The imaging results and the signal cross-spectrum were used to calculate the coherence between all pairings of active cortical locations within each of the 24 frequency bins. Finally, for each active source, the average coherence across frequencies and sources was calculated. In these coherence imaging results (**Fig. 4**), the localization of imaged brain activity strongly depends on the frequency bands with greatest power. **Fig. 4** displays the MEG coherence source imaging (CSI) on the MR imaging axial slices from patient JC287 during a 15-minute resting state with eyes closed. Their arousal level was drowsy to sleeping during this run. JC287 is a 41-year-old right-handed female patient with intractable localization-related epilepsy. Simultaneously recorded EEG found left temporal spikes at electrodes T7>F9>F7, whereas the MEG found spikes in the left hemisphere channels. The single equivalent dipoles mapped 14 spikes (green dipoles) into a focal cluster in the left middle temporal gyrus (**Fig. 5**). The strongest coherent location during this run was found in the left middle temporal gyrus as seen in **Fig. 6**. In this coherence imaging result, the activity is strongest in the 25 to 32 Hz frequency band as well as the 40 to 50 Hz frequency band (**Fig. 7**). A similar study performed by Englot et al found increased coherence in the site of the resection lead to more seizure freedom.[112] Combined DTI and MEG-CSI provided more information on the microstructural changes associated with epileptogenic activity.[113]

Coherence does provide a global estimate of all important regions of network activity regardless of source amplitudes. Because there is a need to minimize bias by increasing the number of data segments in calculations, coherence is not well suited for quantifying rapid temporal changes in synchronized activity. Coherence is best applied to long time series of data to identify sources of brain network activity that persist for long durations. However, it is desirable that the individual FFT components follow temporal changes in network connectivity. Therefore, the length of segments of data used in the FFT transform should be

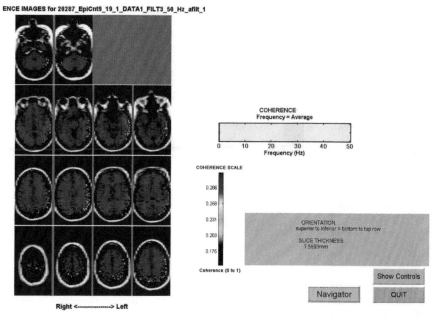

Fig. 4. MEG coherence source imaging (CSI) images overlaid on the axial MR imaging slices for patient JC287. Note that the red areas indicate the highly coherent areas of the brain that were active during this 15-minute resting-state brain scan.

selected in the same way as recommended for correlation calculations. For MEG data the authors have found approximately 0.5 seconds of data to be near optimal for data filtered 3 to 50 Hz. When applied to very low-frequency band data, the FFT data segment length needs to be increased. An F-statistic can be used to test statistical significance relative to the hypothesis of true coherence.[108]

Coherence is best when used for long time series of data to identify sources of brain activity that are part of the same network. Coherence

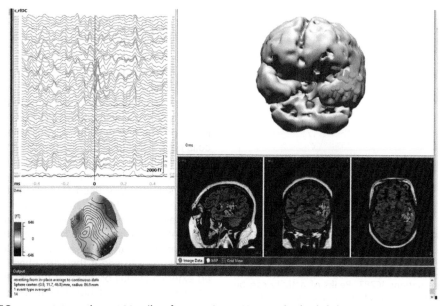

Fig. 5. MEG waves averaged over 14 spikes from patient JC287. Only the left hemisphere MEG channels were selected to perform the dipole fits (*green*) that are shown in the left middle temporal region on the MR imaging slice and on the 3-dimensional cortex.

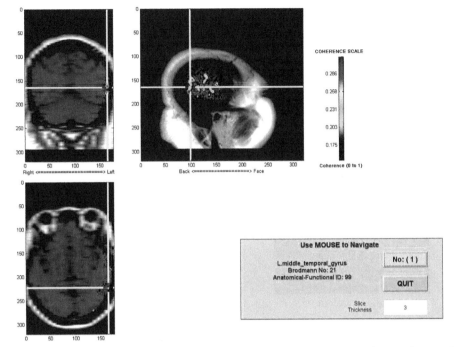

Fig. 6. MEG CSI results of the location that had the highest coherent activity during the 15-minute MEG resting state scan from patient JC287.

analysis supplies information on the degree of synchrony of brain activity at different locations for each frequency, independent of power. However, individual time points with large amplitudes are more highly weighted in the FFT transform

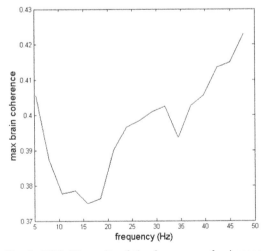

Fig. 7. MEG CSI results of the frequency of coherent activity from patient JC287. Peaks of activity can be seen between 28 and 33 Hz and between 40 and 48 Hz. This corresponds to Fig. 4 and Fig. 6 where the image coherent activity is most likely within these peak frequency bands.

and subsequently in coherence calculations. This is in contrast to phase synchrony, which uses instantaneous measurements of only the phase differences between signals. As mentioned earlier, coherence analysis can be applied to the MEG and EEG waveforms in sensor space or it can be applied to the localized MEG solutions in source space as shown in Fig. 4.

Phase Synchrony

The phase relationship is a way to estimate the synchrony of oscillations in EEG/MEG data. This is the process by which 2 or more electrodes or coils have oscillating activity that are the same or in sync with each other or (in phase) or out of synchrony (out of phase) by a relative phase angle. Phase synchrony is used to investigate whether 2 waveforms with the same narrow frequency band have relatively stable phase differences independent of their amplitude behavior. This is used to determine if the phases are coupled across the brain and to see if they are phase-locked to an external stimuli or event. If the oscillations are all in synchrony and positive at the same time then the phase is 0°, and if they were opposite (one positive and one negative) to each other they would have a phase angle of 180°.[96] Phase synchrony measures how stability of the phase difference varies over a short period of time. Phase relationships can be examined by testing the stability of the signal's phase differences across trials (phase-locking) over a single electrode or between pairs of electrodes.[114] This approach can yield estimates of the precision of local and long-range synchrony. Importantly, measures of phase-locking provide estimates of synchrony independent of the amplitude of oscillations. This is in contrast to measures of coherence where phase and amplitude are intertwined.[115] Phase synchrony reflects the exact timing of communication between distant neural populations that are related functionally, the exchange of information between global and local neuronal networks, and the sequential temporal activity of neural processes in response to incoming sensory stimuli.[116] In the field of schizophrenia Uhlhaas and Singer provided an in-depth review of abnormal neural oscillations and synchrony in this patient group. They review several studies that indicated that patients with schizophrenia have a reduced phase synchrony in the beta and gamma bands.[96]

Phase synchrony is best suited for short duration events such as in an evoked event. Phase is used to determine how much the 2 locations (recording sites) are interacting within a very narrow time window (milliseconds). A great analogy for understanding the difference between when to use coherence or phase synchrony is Soldiers marching in a parade: phase synchrony is used to determine how synchronized their feet are marching in unison in a few steps, whereas coherence is used to see how synchronous their feet were marching in unison over the entire parade route. The results from the analysis of phase synchronization can be used for the quantification of coupling strength and direction because these measures are more sensitive and robust than coherence and phase difference and independent of amplitude dynamics. This is usually applied to a narrow frequency band, usually less then 5 Hz as opposed to a larger frequency range that desynchronizes rapidly due to many varied frequencies mixed in.

SUMMARY

Neurons in the brain communicate by sending oscillating signals along networked pathways in the brain. In this section the authors explain 2 of the most common methods used to analyze the brain's synchronous oscillations as measured with high temporal resolution MEG and/or EEG. They highlight some of the types of information that can be derived from the varied techniques

as well as provide some of the limitations of each technique. In the future a combined anatomic, functional, and effective connectivity mapping will become the mainstay of the neurosurgeon, neurologist, and psychiatrist for assessing and diagnosing normal and abnormal brain networks. These techniques will not only provide biomarkers of diseases but also help to provide individualized treatment therapies based on pre- and posttreatment connectivity imaging. With the evolution of computers and mathematics the authors expect to see more sophisticated and powerful analytical neuroimaging methods developed and applied to the functional neuroimaging data.

DISCLOSURE

The authors have nothing to disclose.

REFERENCES

1. Hämäläinen M, Hari R, Ilmoniemi R, et al. Magnetoencephalography – theory, instrumentation, and applications to noninvasive studies of the working human brain. Rev Mod Phys 1993;65:413–97.
2. Hari R, Ilmoniemi RJ. Cerebral magnetic fields. Crit Rev Biomed Eng 1986;14:93–126.
3. Hämäläinen MS, Sarvas J. Realistic conductivity geometry model of the human head for interpretation of neuromagnetic data. IEEE Trans Biomed Eng 1989;36:165–71.
4. Okada Y, Lahteenmaki A, Xu C. Comparison of MEG and EEG on the basis of somatic evoked responses elicited by stimulation of the snout in the juvenile swine. Clin Neurophysiol 1999;110:214–29.
5. Leahy RM, Mosher JC, Spencer ME, et al. A study of dipole localization accuracy for MEG and EEG using a human skull phantom. Electroencephalogr Clin Neurophysiol 1998;107:159–73.
6. Baillet S, Mosher JC, Leahy RM. Electromagnetic brain mapping. IEEE Signal Process Mag 2001; 18:14–30.
7. Lopes da Silva F, Van Rotterdam A. Biophysical aspects of EEG and MEG generation. In: Niedermeyer E, Lopes da Silva F, editors. Electroencephalography. basic principles, clinical applications and related fields. Baltimore (MD): Lippincott Williams & Wilkins; 1992. p. 91–110.
8. Hämäläinen M, Hari R. Magnetoencephalographic characterization of dynamic brain activation: basic principles and methods of data collection and source analysis. In: Toga AW, Mazziotta JC, editors. Brain mapping, the methods. San Diego (CA): Academic Press; 2002. p. 227–53.
9. Ahlfors SP, Han J, Lin FH, et al. Cancellation of EEG and MEG signals generated by extended and distributed sources. Hum Brain Mapp 2010;31:140–9.

10. Dalal SS, Baillet S, Adam C, et al. Simultaneous MEG and intracranial EEG recordings during attentive reading. NeuroImage 2009;45:1289–304.

11. Tripp JH. Physical concepts and mathematical models. In: Williamson SJ, Romani GL, Kaufman L, et al, editors. Biomagnetism: an interdisciplinary approach. New York: Plenum; 1983. p. 101–39.

12. Kakisaka Y, Kubota Y, Wang ZI, et al. Use of simultaneous depth and MEG recording may provide complementary information regarding the epileptogenic region. Epileptic Disord 2012;14:298–303.

13. Murakami H, Wang ZI, Marashly A, et al. Correlating magnetoencephalography to stereo-electroencephalography in patients undergoing epilepsy surgery. Brain 2016. https://doi.org/10.1093/brain/aww215.

14. Murakami S, Okada Y. Invariance in current dipole moment density across brain structures and species: physiological constraint for neuroimaging. NeuroImage 2015;111:49–58.

15. Goldenholz DM, Ahlfors SP, Hamalainen MS, et al. Mapping the signal-to-noise-ratios of cortical sources in magnetoencephalography and electroencephalography. Hum Brain Mapp 2009;30:1077–86.

16. Plonsey R. Bioelectric phenomena. New York: McGraw-Hill; 1969.

17. Tuch DS, Wedeen VJ, Dale AM, et al. Conductivity tensor mapping of the human brain using diffusion tensor MRI. Proc Natl Acad Sci U S A 2001;98:11697–701.

18. Cuffin BN, Cohen D. Magnetic fields of a dipole in special volume conductor shapes. IEEE Trans Biomed Eng 1977;24:372–81.

19. Ilmoniemi RJ, Hämäläinen MS, Knuutila J. The forward and inverse problems in the spherical model. In: Weinberg H, Stroink G, Katila T, editors. Biomagnetism: applications & theory. New York: Pergamon Press; 1985. p. 278–82.

20. Sarvas J. Basic mathematical and electromagnetic concepts of the biomagnetic inverse problem. Phys Med Biol 1987;32:11–22.

21. Mosher JC, Leahy RM, Lewis PS. EEG and MEG: forward solutions for inverse methods. IEEE Trans Biomed Eng 1999;46:245–59.

22. Stenroos M, Nummenmaa A. Incorporating and compensating cerebrospinal fluid in surface-based forward models of magneto- and electroencephalography. PLoS One 2016;11:e0159595.

23. Stenroos M. Integral equations and boundary-element solution for static potential in a general piece-wise homogeneous volume conductor. Phys Med Biol 2016;61:N606–17.

24. Roche-Labarbe N, Aarabi A, Kongolo G, et al. High-resolution electroencephalography and source localization in neonates. Hum Brain Mapp 2008;29:167–76.

25. Hämäläinen MS, Sarvas J. Feasibility of the homogeneous head model in the interpretation of neuromagnetic fields. Phys Med Biol 1987;32:91–7.

26. Stenroos M, Hunold A, Haueisen J. Comparison of three-shell and simplified volume conductor models in magnetoencephalography. NeuroImage 2014;94:337–48.

27. Huang MX, Song T, Hagler DJ Jr, et al. A novel integrated MEG and EEG analysis method for dipolar sources. Neuroimage 2007;37:731–48.

28. Drechsler F, Wolters CH, Dierkes T, et al. A full subtraction approach for finite element method based source analysis using constrained Delaunay tetrahedralisation. NeuroImage 2009;46:1055–65.

29. Lanfer B, Wolters CH, Demokritov SO, et al. Validating finite element method based EEG and MEG forward computations. Paper presented at the 41 Jahrestagung der Deutschen Gesellschaft für Biomedizinische Technik Aachen. Germany, September 26–29, 2007.

30. Lew S, Sliva DD, Choe MS, et al. Effects of sutures and fontanels on MEG and EEG source analysis in a realistic infant head model. NeuroImage 2013;76C:282–93.

31. Lew S, Wolters CH, Dierkes T, et al. Accuracy and run-time comparison for different potential approaches and iterative solvers in finite element method based EEG source analysis. Appl Numer Math 2009;59:1970–88.

32. Wolters CH, Anwander A, Berti G, et al. Geometry-adapted hexahedral meshes improve accuracy of finite-element-method-based EEG source analysis. IEEE Trans Biomed Eng 2007a;54:1446–53.

33. Wolters CH, Köstler H, Möller C, et al. Numerical approaches for dipole modeling in finite element method based source analysis. Elsevier International Congress Series 2007b;1300:189–92.

34. Wolters CH, Köstler H, Möller C, et al. Numerical mathematics of the subtraction method for the modeling of a current dipole in EEG source reconstruction using finite element head models. SIAM J Sci Comput 2007c;30:24–45.

35. Gullmar D, Haueisen J, Reichenbach JR. Influence of anisotropic electrical conductivity in white matter tissue on the EEG/MEG forward and inverse solution. A high-resolution whole head simulation study. NeuroImage 2010;51:145–63.

36. Dannhauer M, Lanfer B, Wolters CH, et al. Modeling of the human skull in EEG source analysis. Hum Brain Mapp 2011;32:1383–99.

37. Stenroos M, Hauk O. Minimum-norm cortical source estimation in layered head models is robust against skull conductivity error. NeuroImage 2013;81:265–72.

38. Huang M, Aine CJ, Supek S, et al. Multi-start downhill simplex method for spatio-temporal source

localization in magnetoencephalography. Electro-encephalogr Clin Neurophysiol 1998;108:32–44.

39. Mosher JC, Leahy RM. Recursive MUSIC: a framework for EEG and MEG source localization. IEEE Trans Biomed Eng 1998;45:1342–54.

40. Mosher JC, Lewis PS, Leahy RM. Multiple dipole modeling and localization from spatio-temporal MEG data. IEEE Trans Biomed Eng 1992;39: 541–57.

41. Nishitani N, Avikainen S, Hari R. Abnormal imitation-related cortical activation sequences in Asperger's syndrome. Ann Neurol 2004;55:558–62.

42. Salmelin R, Hari R, Lounasmaa OV, et al. Dynamics of brain activation during picture naming. Nature 1994;368:463–5.

43. Salmelin R, Hari R. Spatiotemporal characteristics of sensorimotor neuromagnetic rhythms related to thumb movement. Neuroscience 1994;60:537–50.

44. Dale AM, Liu AK, Fischl BR, et al. Dynamic statistical parametric mapping: combining fMRI and MEG for high-resolution imaging of cortical activity. Neuron 2000;26:55–67.

45. Dale AM, Sereno MI. Improved localization of cortical activity by combining EEG and MEG with MRI cortical surface reconstruction: A linear approach. J Cogn Neurosci 1993;5:162–76.

46. Hämäläinen M, Ilmoniemi R. Interpreting magnetic fields of the brain: minimum norm estimates. Espoo (Finland): Helsinki University of Technology; 1984.

47. Uutela K, Hämäläinen M, Somersalo E. Visualization of magnetoencephalographic data using minimum current estimates. NeuroImage 1999;10:173–80.

48. Gramfort A, Kowalski M, Hamalainen M. Mixed-norm estimates for the M/EEG inverse problem using accelerated gradient methods. Phys Med Biol 2012;57:1937–61.

49. Gramfort A, Strohmeier D, Haueisen J, et al. Time-frequency mixed-norm estimates: sparse M/EEG imaging with non-stationary source activations. NeuroImage 2013;70:410–22.

50. Ou W, Hamalainen MS, Golland P. A distributed spatio-temporal EEG/MEG inverse solver. NeuroImage 2009;44:932–46.

51. Ioannides AA, Liu MJ, Liu LC, et al. Magnetic field tomography of cortical and deep processes: examples of "real-time mapping" of averaged and single trial MEG signals. Int J Psychophysiol 1995;20: 161–75.

52. Moran JE, Bowyer S, Tepley N. Multi-Resolution FOCUSS: a source imaging technique applied to MEG data. Brain Topogr 2005;18:1–17.

53. Huang MX, Dale AM, Song T, et al. Vector-based spatial-temporal minimum L1-norm solution for MEG. Neuroimage 2006;31:1025–37.

54. Huang MX, Huang CW, Robb A, et al. MEG source imaging method using fast L1 minimum-norm and its applications to signals with brain noise and human resting-state source amplitude images. Neuroimage 2014;84:585–604.

55. Sekihara K, Nagarajan SS. Adaptive spatial filters for electromagnetic brain imaging. Berlin, Heidelberg: Springer-Verlag; 2008.

56. Van Veen B, Buckley K. Beamforming: a versatile approach to spatial filtering. IEEE assp magazine 1988.

57. Steinstrater O, Sillekens S, Junghoefer M, et al. Sensitivity of beamformer source analysis to deficiencies in forward modeling. Hum Brain Mapp 2010;31:1907–27.

58. Tanaka N, Hämäläinen MS, Ahlfors SP, et al. Propagation of epileptic spikes reconstructed from spatiotemporal magnetoencephalographic and electroencephalographic source analysis. NeuroImage 2010;50:217–22.

59. Jones EG. Viewpoint: the core and matrix of thalamic organization. Neuroscience 1998;85: 331–45.

60. Jones EG. The thalamic matrix and thalamocortical synchrony. Trends Neurosci 2001;24:595–601.

61. Steriade M, McCormick DA, Sejnowski TJ. Thalamocortical oscillations in the sleeping and aroused brain. Science 1993;262:679–85.

62. Alexander GE, DeLong MR, Strick PL. Parallel organization of functionally segregated circuits linking basal ganglia and cortex. Annu Rev Neurosci 1986;9:357–81.

63. Graybiel AM. The basal ganglia. Curr Biol 2000;10: R509–11.

64. Phelps EA, LeDoux JE. Contributions of the amygdala to emotion processing: from animal models to human behavior. Neuron 2005;48:175–87.

65. Krishnaswamy P, Obregon-Henao G, Ahveninen J, et al. Sparsity enables estimation of both subcortical and cortical activity from MEG and EEG. Proc Natl Acad Sci U S A 2017;114:E10465–74.

66. Babadi B, Obregon-Henao G, Lamus C, et al. A Subspace Pursuit-based Iterative Greedy Hierarchical solution to the neuromagnetic inverse problem. NeuroImage 2014;87:427–43.

67. Huang CW, Huang M-X, Ji Z, et al. High-resolution MEG source imaging approach to accurately localize Broca's area in patients with brain tumor or epilepsy. Clin Neurophysiol 2016;127:2308–16.

68. Kandel ER, Schwartz JH, Jessell TM, et al. Principles of neural science. 5th edition. New York: McGraw-Hill Companies, Inc.; 2013.

69. Hari R, Forss N. Magnetoencephalography in the study of human somatosensory cortical processing. Philos Trans R Soc Lond B Biol Sci 1999;354: 1145–54.

70. Hari R, Karhu J, Hamalainen M, et al. Functional organization of the human first and second somatosensory cortices: a neuromagnetic study. Eur J Neurosci 1993;5:724–34.

71. Huang MX, Lee RR, Miller GA, et al. A parietal-frontal network studied by somatosensory oddball MEG responses, and its cross-modal consistency. NeuroImage 2005;28:99–114.

72. Simoes C, Jensen O, Parkkonen L, et al. Phase locking between human primary and secondary somatosensory cortices. Proc Natl Acad Sci U S A 2003;100:2691–4.

73. Huang M-X, Nichols S, Baker DG, et al. Single-subject-based whole-brain MEG slow-wave imaging approach for detecting abnormality in patients with mild traumatic brain injury. Neuroimage Clin 2014b;5:109–19.

74. Huang M-X, Nichols S, Robb A, et al. An automatic MEG low-frequency source imaging approach for detecting injuries in mild and moderate TBI patients with blast and non-blast causes. NeuroImage 2012;61:1067–82.

75. Huang M-X, Yurgil KA, Robb A, et al. Voxel-wise resting-state MEG source magnitude imaging study reveals neurocircuitry abnormality in active-duty service members and veterans with PTSD. Neuroimage Clin 2014c;5:408–19.

76. Berger H. Uber das Elektrenkephalogramm des Menschen. Arch Psychiatr Nervenkr 1929;87:527–70.

77. Cohen D. Detection of magnetic fields outside the human head produced by alpha rhythm currents. Electroencephalogr Clin Neurophysiol 1970;28:102.

78. Cohen D. Magnetoencephalography: evidence of magnetic fields produced by alpha-rhythm currents. Science 1968;161:784–6.

79. Hari R, Salmelin R, Makela JP, et al. Magnetoencephalographic cortical rhythms. Int J Psychophysiol 1997;26:51–62.

80. Niedermeyer E, Lopes da Silva FH. Electroencephalography: basic principles, clinical applications, and related fields. Philadelphia: Lippincott Williams & Wilkins; 2005.

81. Manshanden I, De Munck JC, Simon NR, et al. Source localization of MEG sleep spindles and the relation to sources of alpha band rhythms. ClinNeurophysiol 2002;113:1937–47.

82. Mizuki Y, Kajimura N, Kai S, et al. Differential responses to mental stress in high and low anxious normal humans assessed by frontal midline theta activity. Int J Psychophysiol 1992;12:169–78.

83. Mizuki Y, Kajimura N, Nishikori S, et al. Appearance of frontal midline theta rhythm and personality traits. Folia Psychiatr Neurol Jpn 1984;38:451–8.

84. Mizuki Y, Tanaka M, Isozaki H, et al. Periodic appearance of theta rhythm in the frontal midline area during performance of a mental task. Electroencephalogr Clin Neurophysiol 1980;49:345–51.

85. Takahashi N, Shinomiya S, Mori D, et al. Frontal midline theta rhythm in young healthy adults. Clin Electroencephalogr 1997;28:49–54.

86. Fries P. Rhythms for cognition: communication through coherence. Neuron 2015;88:220–35.

87. Tewarie P, Liuzzi L, O'Neill GC, et al. Tracking dynamic brain networks using high temporal resolution MEG measures of functional connectivity. Neuroimage 2019;200:38–50.

88. Friston KJ, Frith CD, Liddle PF, et al. Functional connectivity: the principal-component analysis of large (PET) data sets. J Cereb BloodFlow Metab 1993;13:5–14.

89. Greenblatt RE, Pflieger ME, Ossadtchi AE. Connectivity measures applied to human brain electrophysiological data. J Neurosci Methods 2012;2007(1):1–16.

90. Sakkalis V. Review of advanced techniques for the estimation of brain connectivity measured with EEG/MEG. Comput Biol Med 2011;41:1110–7.

91. Lehnertz K, Mormann F, Osterhage H, et al. State-of-the-art of seizure prediction. J Clin Neurophysiol 2007;24(2):147–53.

92. Bastos AM, Schoffelen J-M. A tutorial review of functional connectivity analysis methods and their interpretational pitfalls. Front Syst Neurosci 2016;9:175.

93. Cabral J, Kringelbach ML, Deco G. Exploring the network dynamics underlying brain activity during rest. Prog Neurobiol 2014;114:102–31.

94. Towle VL, Hunter JD, Edgar JC, et al. Frequency domain analysis of human subdural recordings. J Clin Neurophysiol 2007;24(2):205–13.

95. Hinkley LB, Vinogradov S, Guggisberg AG, et al. Clinical symptoms and alpha band resting-state functional connectivity imaging in patients with schizophrenia: implications for novel approaches to treatment. Biol Psychiatry 2011;70(12):1134–42.

96. Uhlhaas PJ, Singer W. Abnormal neural oscillations and synchrony in schizophrenia. Nat Rev Neurosci 2010;11(2):100–13.

97. Chana G, Bousman CA, Money TT, et al. Biomarker investigations related to pathophysiological pathways in schizophrenia and psychosis. Front Cell Neurosci 2013;7(95):1–18.

98. Llinas RR. The Intrinsic electrophysiological properties of mammalian neurons: a new insight into CNS function. Science 1988;242(4886):1654–64.

99. Llinas RR, Grace AA, Yarom Y. In vitro neurons in mammalian cortical layer 4 exhibit intrinsic oscillatory activity in the 10- to 50-Hz frequency range. Proc Natl Acad Sci U S A 1991;88(3):897–901.

100. Haenschel C, Linden D. Exploring intermediate phenotypes with eeg: working memory dysfunction in schizophrenia. Behav Brain Res 2011;216:481–95.

101. Stephan KE, Friston KJ, Frith C. Dysconnection in schizophrenia: From abnormal synaptic plasticity to failures of self-monitoring. Schizophr Bull 2009;35:509–27.

102. Wang XJ. Neurophysiological and computational principles of cortical rhythms in cognition. Physiol Rev 2010;90:1195–268.

103. Ogawa S, Lee TM, Kay AR, et al. Brain magnetic resonance imaging with contrast dependent on blood oxygenation. Proc Natl Acad Sci US A 1990;87:9868–72.

104. Varela F, Lachaux JP, Rodriguez E, et al. The brain-web: phase synchronization and large-scale integration. Nat Rev Neurosci 2001;2(4):229–39.

105. Horwitz B. The elusive concept of brain connectivity. NeuroImage 2003;19:466–70.

106. Gross J, Timmermann L, Kujala J, et al. The neural basis of intermittent motor control in humans. Proc Natl Acad Sci U S A 2002;99(4):2299–302.

107. French CC, Beaumont JG. A critical review of EEG coherence studies of hemisphere function. Int J Psychophysiol 1984;1(3):241–54.

108. Kelly EF, Lenz JE, Franaszczk PJ, et al. A general statistical framework for frequency-domain analysis of EEG topographic structure. Comput Biomed Res 1997;30:129–64.

109. Song J, Tucker DM, Gilbert T, et al. Methods for examining electrophysiological coherence in epileptic networks. Front Neurol 2013;4:55.

110. Elisevich K, Shukla N, Moran JE, et al. An assessment of MEG coherence imaging in the study of temporal lobe epilepsy. Epilepsia 2011;52(6):1110–9.

111. Moran JE, Drake CL, Tepley N. ICA methods for MEG imaging. Neurol Clin Neurophysiol 2004;2004:72.

112. Englot DJ, Hinkley LB, Kort NS, et al. Global and regional functional connectivity maps of neural oscillations in focal epilepsy. Brain 2015;138(Pt 8):2249–62.

113. Nazem-Zadeh MR, Bowyer SM, Moran JE, et al. MEG Coherence and DTI Connectivity in mTLE. Brain Topogr 2016;29(4):598–622.

114. Lachaux JP, Rodriguez E, Martinerie J, et al. Measuring phase synchrony in brain signals. Hum Brain Mapp 1999;8:194–208.

115. Uhlhaas PJ, Roux F, Rodriguez E, et al. Neural synchrony and the development of cortical networks. Trends Cogn Sci 2009;14(2):72–80.

116. Sauseng P, Klimesch W. What does phase information of oscillatory brain activity tell us about cognitive processes? Neurosci Biobehav Rev 2008;32(5):1001–13.

MEG for Greater Sensitivity and More Precise Localization in Epilepsy

Richard C. Burgess, MD, PhD

KEYWORDS

- Magnetoencephalography • Magnetic source imaging • Source localization • Source model
- Head model • Dipole • Magnetometer • Gradiometer

KEY POINTS

- Although sometimes referred to as "magnetic source imaging," MEG is a clinical neurophysiology tool (like EEG), not an imaging method. Like EEG, MEG has excellent temporal resolution.
- Compared to EEG, MEG has superior spatial resolution, because the recorded magnetic signals are not attenuated or influenced by the intervening layers of CSF, bone, or scalp.
- Sources of epileptic activity are localized using computer models of the source and of the head to solve the "inverse problem."
- Like EEG, there are artifacts and normal variants (many are unique to MEG) which must be excluded or recognized; this takes considerable skill and experience.

The magnetic equivalent of electroencephalography (EEG), magnetoencephalography (MEG) is a direct electrophysiologic measure of neural function that records the magnetic fields just outside the scalp on a millisecond-by-millisecond basis. MEG is based on recording these incredibly small magnetic fields, typically tens to hundreds of femtotesla (10^{-14} to 10^{-13} T), noninvasively. The data collected during MEG recording are processed at the completion of the test using mathematical modeling to determine the location, strength, and orientation of the currents producing the magnetic field. Because the MEG helmet into which the patients are introduced has hundreds of sensors, and the magnetic field is not distorted by skull or other boundaries, this modality has greater localization accuracy than EEG and indicates more precisely where neural activity is originating. This good spatial resolution is coupled with superb time resolution, so propagation and aberrant conduction of epileptic activity can be assessed in detail.

The basic modalities of MEG with approved clinical indications are:

- Spontaneous MEG for identification of epileptic foci
- Presurgical mapping of eloquent cortex (usually before resection of a mass lesion)

MEG is highly accurate for the localization of epileptiform discharges and can be used to direct the surgical strategy or to help optimize the rest of the evaluation. Presurgical mapping in epilepsy is designed to minimize or avoid a postoperative deficit. The goals are a bit different in cases of tumoral surgery or other mass lesion resection, where the surgery is designed to prolong survival, and the presurgical mapping helps to optimize the trade-off with postoperative quality of life.

In the population of patients with epilepsy (the main focus of this article), MEG is used to localize interictal spikes, to guide further evaluation (eg, placement of invasive electrodes), and to outline the precise relationship of the epileptogenic zone to a known lesion. It helps to mediate between other discordant diagnostic tests, especially in nonlesional patients, and can suggest that a

Published previously in Clinical Neurophysiology: Basis and Technical Aspects, Volume 160, 1st Edition.
Epilepsy Center, Neurological Institute, The Cleveland Clinic Foundation, 9500 Euclid Avenue, Cleveland, OH 44195, USA
E-mail address: burgesr@ccf.org

neuroimaging.theclinics.com

patient with apparently generalized epilepsy actually has a focus that should be further investigated for possible resection. It can uncover or confirm additional foci, thereby eliminating the patient from consideration as a possible surgical candidate, and can detect epileptiform activity when the EEG is normal or equivocal.

Multiple studies have demonstrated the clinical value of MEG. These studies include demonstration that MEG provides additional localizing information,[1,2] that the results of MEG change electrode coverage decisions for intracranial EEG, and that the yield of MEG is higher than that from scalp EEG.[3,4]

In patients with epilepsy, MEG is always carried out with simultaneous recording of EEG, to identify via MEG the patient's habitual interictal and ictal abnormalities, and also to see the origin and propagation of the epileptic focus as it spreads sufficiently to be seen on EEG.

COMPARISON WITH THE ELECTROENCEPHALOGRAM

Especially important in epilepsy, MEG has a higher signal-to-noise ratio (SNR) than an EEG, and a higher detection sensitivity for interictal discharges. Compared with simultaneous EEG, the yield of epileptic abnormalities in MEG recordings of spontaneous brain activity is higher.[3] MEG's sensitivity advantage compared with EEG has also been demonstrated in simultaneous

MEG and intracranial EEG recordings where the amount of cortex that needed to be activated to produce a spike identifiable in MEG was 3 to 4 cm^2.[5] Although an early in vitro study claimed that as little as 6 cm^2 of activated gyral cortex could result in an EEG spike,[6] a later in vivo investigation found that 10 cm^2 or more of discharging cortex was needed to produce a scalp spike that was notable above background EEG, and that many prominent EEG spikes had generator areas of 20 to 30 cm^2.[7] Therefore, MEG can pick up activity from cortical areas that are 3 to 10 times smaller than scalp EEG. **Fig. 1** shows an example of the higher sensitivity of MEG.

Although it is the magnetic equivalent of EEG, MEG has several advantages over EEG:

1. It has an inherently higher source resolution.
2. Recordings are reference free.
3. Because the magnetic susceptibility is the same for all the tissues (including the skull), MEG signals are not attenuated by bone and scalp, and therefore the signals are not distorted as they pass from inside the head to the external magnetic sensors.
4. It is easy to obtain multichannel (100–300 channels), whole-head, high spatial density, wideband (DC–2000 Hz) recordings.

Thus, MEG allows for a more accurate measurement and localization of brain activities, importantly epileptic abnormalities.

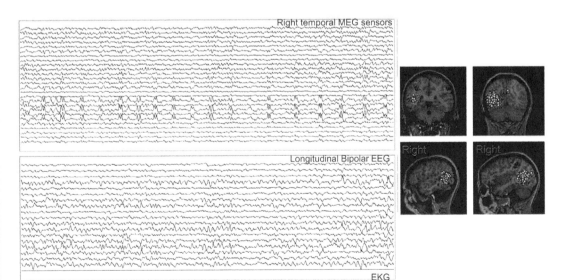

Fig. 1. Note the repetitive periodic lateralized epileptiform discharges (PLED)-like discharges seen in the right temporal MEG sensors (*top*). This activity is not visible in the simultaneous EEG (*bottom*, longitudinal bipolar montage). Source localization showed a tight cluster in the right temporal–parietal–occipital junction (*right*).

INTEGRATION OF MAGNETOENCEPHALOGRAPHY INTO THE EVALUATION OF PATIENTS WITH EPILEPSY

Methods for imaging the brain fall into structural (or anatomic) imaging and functional imaging. Computed tomography scans and MR images are examples of structural imaging, whereas PET and functional MR images are examples of functional imaging. Whereas other modalities infer brain function indirectly by measuring changes in blood flow, metabolism, oxygenation, and so on, MEG, together with EEG, measures neuronal and synaptic function directly. Fusing (coregistering) the results of structural and functional imaging offers the opportunity for precise localization of neurologic physiology—or pathophysiology. MEG is also known as magnetic source imaging, and although the results are coregistered to show the locations of brain activity sources in 3 dimensions, it is fundamentally a clinical neurophysiologic test, like EEG.

Recording and analysis of brain activity as a function of time has been the province of the EEG and Evoked Potentials, EPs. EEG and evoked potentials are recordings of the electrical activity of neurons; they seem to be similar to an EKG, except that they require many (often hundreds of) channels or traces. Like an EEG, a MEG records a multichannel amplitude versus time representation of brain activity (**Fig. 2**). Because MEG shares with EEG millisecond time resolution, it is much more sensitive to rapid

changes in brain activity (such as those that occur during seizure propagation) than PET or single photon emission computed tomography. **Fig. 3** illustrates MEG's ability to discern rapid propagation of epileptic activity.

Magnetoencephalography Instrumentation

The tiny magnetic fields generated by the neuronal currents induce an electric current in detection coils that are rendered superconducting by immersion in liquid helium. These coils are arrayed within a helmet-shaped dewar (a liquid helium container vessel) that surrounds the head.[8,9] Each of the several hundred coils is immersed in liquid helium, maintained at a temperature of 4.2°K, and coupled to a superconducting quantum interference device that produces an output voltage proportional to the magnetic field.

Because the magnetic fields produced by the brain are so small in comparison with other magnetic noise in the environment, they are difficult to record without some kind of shielding. MEG recording is carried out inside a magnetically shielded room to attenuate the effects of external sources of magnetic noise, such as moving vehicles, elevators, machinery, powerlines, and so on, which are often 6 orders of magnitude larger than the fields produced by the brain.

Because they must be cooled down close to absolute zero, the magnetic sensors cannot be placed on the head. Therefore, unlike EEG where the electrodes are in fixed positions on the scalp,

EEG and MEG waveforms

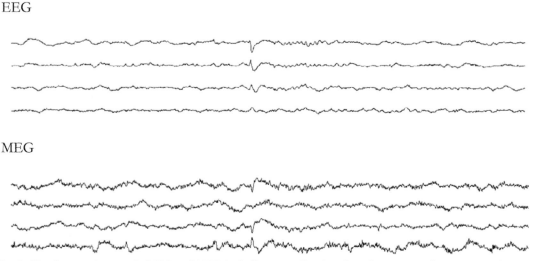

Fig. 2. Simultaneously recorded EEG and MEG, including an epileptic spike. The 8-s page demonstrates the similarity of the waveforms, which both derive from the same underlying neuronal currents.

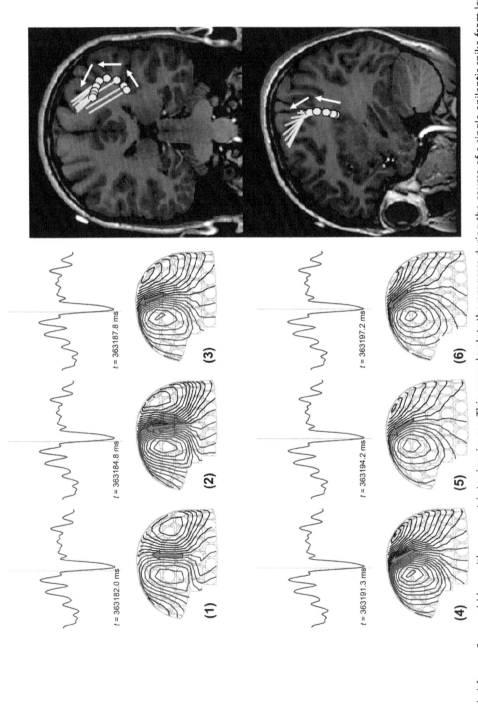

Fig. 3. Recorded from a 9-year-old boy with asymmetric tonic seizures. This example plots the progress during the course of a single epileptic spike from left supramarginal to left precentral over 20 ms in the coronal and sagittal MR imaging views. This propagation track was produced by sequentially fitting a single equivalent dipole at intervals of 1 ms. Magnetic field plots at 3-m intervals are shown on the left, with gradient lines in red denoting magnetic efflux and blue indicating influx. The patient subsequently underwent resection of a focal dysplasia from the initial location shown by MEG.

the physical relationship of the sensors to the scalp—and to the underlying cortex—is not fixed and must be measured for each patient. In addition, the location of the head within the dewar varies from patient to patient, and it changes even during a recording session on an individual patient.

The spatial relationships of the sensor locations to the brain are obtained indirectly based on 3-dimensional digitization of several anatomic landmarks, such as nasion and preauricular points, and by head position indicating (HPI) coils, so that their positions can be coregistered with the same landmarks ascertained from the patient's MR imaging study. The measurement that establishes the relationship of the head to the sensors is done by generating known magnetic fields in a few[10–12] small HPI coils that are affixed to the scalp. The locations of the HPI coils on the head are, in turn, established before the patient enters the shielded room, usually with a wand-like device (which in most systems also uses magnetic field localization principles).

Using the locations of HPI coils measured on the scalp, the MEG sensor space is coregistered to the patient's own MR imaging space so that activity arising from any 3-dimensional location within the helmet can be shown in MR imaging space, to within a coregistration accuracy of 3 to 4 mm. In the most modern MEG systems, the patient's head position within the helmet is not only established at the beginning of the test, but is tracked continuously (this so-called continuous HPI typically runs at 100 times per second).

The configuration of the whole-head sensor systems (Fig. 4) and the associated acquisition hardware enables high-density (200–300 channels), wideband (DC–2000 Hz) recordings of currents within the brain. Detailed minimal standards for clinical MEG have been published by the American Clinical MEG Society.

MAGNETOENCEPHALOGRAPHY RECORDING

Because the patient must remain relatively still during a MEG recording, duration is limited and generally confined to the interictal state.[13] Typical MEG monitoring times for patients with epilepsy range from 40 minutes to a few hours. Continuous head position monitoring and correction allow the patient modest freedom of movement and obviate the need for general anesthesia. These systems that can continuously monitor and correct for head movement are well-developed and clinically validated.[14] Incorporation of these movement compensation methods into commercial MEG systems has dramatically increased their practical clinical usefulness, especially in very young children who are unable to stay still,[15] and MEG is now extensively used in children.[16–22]

The procedure for MEG recording consists of the following steps:

- Attachment of scalp EEG electrodes using the customary international 10 to 20 electrode positions.
- Attachment of HPI coils.
- Digitization of fiducials (typically nasion and preauricular points) to orient the head with respect to MR imaging.
- Digitization of a cloud of scalp points to permit coregistration with surface reconstruction of the MR imaging.
- Demagnetization of the patient with a hand-held degausser.
- Placement of the patient's head inside the dewar containing the sensor array and verification of satisfactory initial placement (Fig. 5).
- Recording of signals from the HPI coils to establish their location inside the array, with continuous HPI coil monitoring where available.
- Acquisition of MEG signals for the duration of the recording session, with the data usually broken into reasonably sized data epochs for ease of data handling.
- Continue recording long enough to capture adequate samples of abnormal discharges (typically 1 hour).
- Data analysis, including review of simultaneous video (especially for ictal MEGs) and contemporaneously placed annotations/markers.
- Source localization of the abnormal waveforms identified.

MEG instrumentation

•SQUID

•Flux transformers

•Shielded room

•Head position indicator

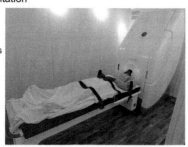

Fig. 4. Patients may be recorded in a supine or seated position. The gantry contains a cylindrical dewar with a helmet-shaped concavity on one end, into which the subject's head is placed for measurement. Liquid helium inside the dewar maintains superconductivity of the pickup coils (magnetometers and/or gradiometers).

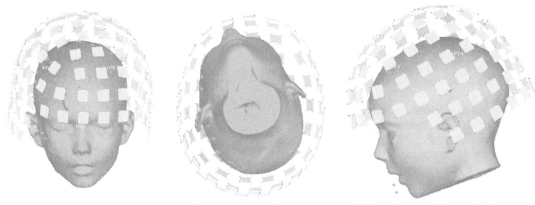

Fig. 5. A display shows the alignment of the subject in the MEG array. Full insertion provides optimal coverage and good signal quality. Head position is monitored continuously (cHPI) by coils affixed to the scalp.

The digitization of the points on the head before placing the patient in the magnetically shielded room can be done with a magnetic stylus, a laser wand, or a video/photographic target device, depending on the manufacturer.

PEDIATRIC MAGNETOENCEPHALOGRAPHY

Although many of our young patients with epilepsy have generalized disorders and are therefore not good candidates for epilepsy surgery, the superior temporal and spatial resolution of MEG can reveal focal regions of epileptogenicity, thereby altering treatment. The most commonly appreciated challenges to infant MEG are[23] the signal attenuation associated with increased scalp-to-sensor distance and[24] the artifact and location uncertainty created by patient movement. Because the patients are so young, they are unable to follow instructions to remain still, and the smaller size of their heads means that they have considerable range of movement within the relatively large sensor helmet of the whole head MEG systems available today.

Technological advances in MEG have ameliorated the problems accompanying infant recordings, and laboratories have adopted procedures to optimize the recording environment and signal quality:

- Postprocessing to separate noise sources and eliminate artifact
- Continuous head position monitoring and movement compensation
- Procedures for comforting the baby and optimizing recordings

These and other improvements have made it possible to record satisfactory MEGs in infants using the conventional adult apparatus, with findings that inform the therapeutic decision even more frequently than in adults.[15,25]

ANALYSIS, SOURCE LOCALIZATION, AND INTERPRETATION OF MAGNETOENCEPHALOGRAMS

The origin of the electrical currents in the brain must be inferred from the extracranial electric potentials (EEG) or magnetic field (MEG), based on a projection of extracranial field data onto the surface or into the volume of the brain. MEG source estimation is unfortunately an ill-posed inverse problem, which depends on modeling the source and the head. The most common methods for solving this inverse problem use parametric approaches, in clinical practice typically using the single equivalent current dipole (SECD) to model the source.[26] There are multipolar models, as well as linear imaging methods (using boundary element models or finite element models to model the head), but the SECD is practical and accurate for focal sources.

A current dipole generated in the cerebral cortex produces not only electric potentials, but also magnetic field. To locate the generators requires modeling of the source, that is, estimation of the current distribution inside the brain from the measured magnetic field distribution. This problem, called the inverse problem, is inherently ill-posed and therefore does not have a unique solution, but it can be approached by imposing some reasonable constraints. The SECD model is frequently used because it is both accurate and practical. We compare the measured and the modeled field distributions by iteratively testing the fields that would be generated from a source with a known location and orientation, that is, the forward problem, which does have a unique solution based on Maxwell's equations. Because the electrical activities on the scalp are affected by neighboring brain structures and lack of tissue homogeneity, and the corresponding magnetic fields are not, the calculations required to deduce the source are considerably simpler for MEG than for EEG signals. The SECD is not a perfect representation for all brain activity, but is a good model for activity that involves a few square centimeters of cortex.

As with MEG, it is possible to fruitfully carry out source localization of EEG activity,[27] and the results of MEG and EEG source localization are complementary.[28] In conventional clinical practice, only 20 to 30 scalp electrodes are typically used, whereas whole-head MEG systems all include several hundred sensors. It has been shown that a greater number of EEG channels than the traditional international 10 to 20, for example, 64 to 128 or more, improves the identification and source models of EEG spikes.[29] Whole-head MEG systems currently have an accuracy of 3 to 4 mm when dipolar sources with an adequate SNR are localized, whereas an EEG does no better than 7 to 8 mm, even when higher density EEG placement is used.

Along with its strength, the orientation of the cortical source (primarily the orientation of the pyramidal cells) determines the degree to which a magnetic field is externally observed. Although fundamental physics principles dictate that MEG cannot detect magnetic fields arising from currents with a radial orientation, and therefore is theoretically blind to the activity of sources in the gyral crowns, it is extremely rare not to see activity on MEG that is picked up by EEG. As noted elsewhere in this article, the sensitivity of MEG is in fact considerably greater than that of EEG. After the sources of the magnetic fields have been mapped in 3-dimensional space, they can be coregistered with and displayed on the patient's MR imaging (**Fig. 6**).

Reliable localization of an epileptic source generally requires that at least 5 spikes are found in the same region.[10–12] When 5 or even more spikes cluster within the same sublobar region and have a constant orientation, this consistency increases confidence that the localization accurately depicts the epileptogenic zone, as shown by the example in **Fig. 7**. The degree to which a group of locations shows sufficient adjacency to be called a cluster varies across MEG centers,[5,19,30–33] but a useful objective characterization of the cluster size and orientation cone can be derived from a *k*-means partitioning method.[24] It is important to remember that the accuracy of source localization is highly dependent on the SNR of the spikes. A low SNR produces a

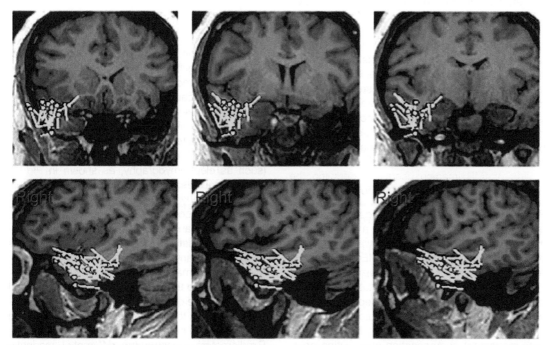

Fig. 6. With the patient's position inside the array monitored and the localization of the magnetic sources within the array, the sources can be coregistered to the patient's MR imaging. The *yellow circles* each indicate the location of an epileptic spike in the right anterior temporal region, and the *yellow tails* show the orientation of the sources.

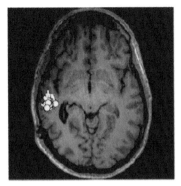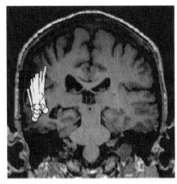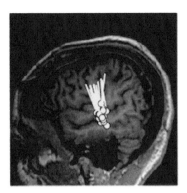

Fig. 7. In this example, many epileptic spikes were recorded from the right temporal lobe during the MEG. The spike localization results demonstrate tightly clustered equivalent current dipole sources with consistent vertical orientation. Highly repeatable results from spike to spike, as in this patient, reinforce the accuracy of localization.

scattered appearance, even when the sources are identically located.[34] For this reason, some magnetoencephalographers prefer to carry out spike averaging before source localization to achieve adequate SNR.[28,35,36] Averaging itself has its own perils, however, in that it depends on the identicalness of each of the spikes in the ensemble, and it obscures location differences that may be of clinical importance,[37,38] such as sources arising from opposite sides of a sulcus. Fortunately, the acceptability of the localization results for an individual spike can be determined from the magnetic field pattern and the ECD statistics.[39] Because of its better resolution compared with scalp EEG, MEG is often able to resolve what seem to be hemispheric discharges on EEG into multiple separate clusters on MEG[40,41]—which has important ramifications for clinical decision making.[42] Although some epileptogenic regions that are too small or too distant from the sensors are not detected by MEG[43,44] until some spread to larger regions has occurred, clusters of sources localized from clearly epileptic activity should not be ignored,[45] even if discordant with other modalities.[46]

ICTAL MAGNETOENCEPHALOGRAPHY

Because it is difficult for patients to remain still for extended periods of time, MEG mainly records interictal spikes. There are, however, patients who have seizures during their MEG recordings, either because of the very high seizure frequency in some patients with intractable epilepsy, because they have been sleep deprived or activated, or simply because of serendipity. In our laboratory, this happens in more than 10% of cases. With movement compensation and routine postprocessing, MEG signals at the seizure onset are of good quality, and accurate localization of the ictal sources can be achieved.[14]

In a recent study[23] of the information provided by ictal MEG, 44 patients out of 377 consecutive MEG studies had seizures recorded during their MEG (12% of the patients with refractory epilepsy referred to the MEG laboratory). Analysis was limited by patient movement in only 3 of the cases. When both ictal and interictal abnormalities were recorded, dipole localizations showed a high concordance. The MEG seizures showed a more focal onset than EEG, and in 16 cases (36%) provided localizing information not available on EEG. There were 8 cases (18.1%) where ictal MEG provided unique findings not detected interictally.

ARTIFACTS IN MAGNETOENCEPHALOGRAPHY

Artifacts are the bane of the existence of clinical neurophysiologists. The usual problems that plague EEG, such as movement, external electrical apparatus, electrocardiogram, and electromyogram, are also factors in MEG. Although MEG necessitates a shielded room for recording, interfering signals are not altogether worse than in EEG, but rather they are different. In fact, some artifacts (such as electromyography, as shown in **Fig. 8**) are less troublesome in MEG. As in other areas of clinical neurophysiology, the main principles of prevention and recognition are primary. Furthermore, active noise cancellation, that is, real-time feedback compensation using active field coils, helps to counteract any residual interference that penetrates into the magnetically shielded room.

Analogous to the familiar bipolar montages used in EEG, the use of gradiometers instead of magnetometers helps to cancel out noise common to the 2 coils that are carrying out the signal subtraction. Gradiometers measure the differential magnetic fields coupled to the superconducting quantum interference devices. Implanted devices such as vagal nerve stimulators, pacemakers, and

EEG

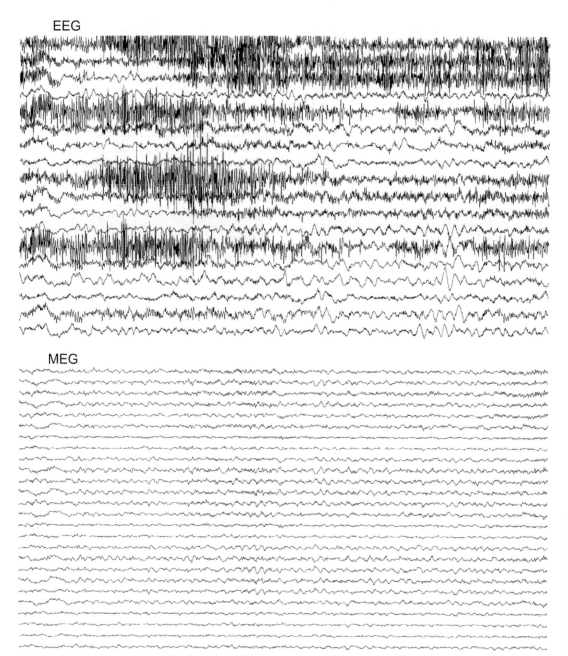

MEG

Fig. 8. Ten-second page of EEG (*top*) and simultaneously recorded MEG (*bottom*). Noise reduction techniques discriminate against signals that are not coming from inside the head. Notice that the EEG is contaminated with considerable electromyographic artifact, while the MEG is immune to the extracranial sources.

responsive neural stimulators do not preclude MEG recording, but postprocessing to eliminate extracranial interference is required (eg, spatiotemporal signal space separation[47]).

NORMAL VARIANTS IN MAGNETOENCEPHALOGRAPHY

Like EEG, there is a certain amount of art to MEG interpretation—despite the sophistication of MEG hardware and its considerably greater dependence on computer methods. A normal variant is a suspicious waveform that mimics something else, but is within the range of normal activity. Not all normal MEG variants have EEG counterparts, and several have an epileptiform appearance. Misidentification of these physiologic transients can lead to inappropriate further diagnostic testing, or even to harmful treatment decisions.[48] The results of MEG are

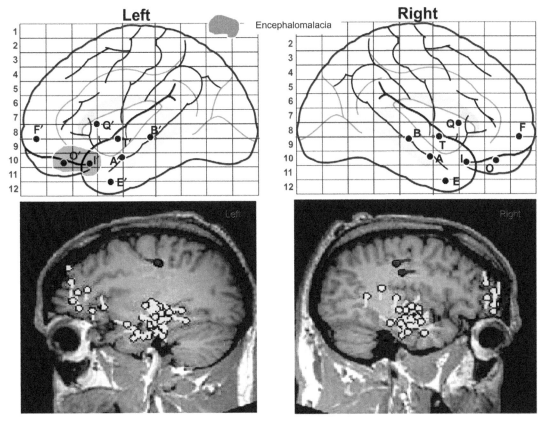

Fig. 9. Preimplantation map, planning locations for SEEG insertion, based substantially on the MEG localization of the epileptic sources. One of the primary indications for MEG in complicated epilepsy cases is for guidance of intracranial electrode placement.

used to plan the implantation of intracranial electrodes (**Fig. 9**) or to define a resective strategy. Sources highlighted on MEG guide the surgeon, and therefore it is important that all the identified sources are truly epileptic.

Normal variants seen in MEG can be divided into (1) those that correspond to well-known normal EEG variants (such as small sharp spikes (BETS), POSTS, vertex transients, etc) and (2) those discharges that are only seen on MEG and that have no EEG counterpart (such as supramarginal transients, and perirolandic transients).

These MEG-specific transients are almost always MEG unique; that is, they are not seen on the simultaneously recorded EEG channels. Of course, there are physiologic variants in EEG that have no MEG counterpart, such as spiky appearing breach rhythms. Because MEG has no vulnerability to the conductivity differences associated with a neurosurgical or traumatic breach, the MEG waveform is not affected. By the same token, not all MEG-unique transients are normal variants. Because the yield of MEG for truly epileptic spikes is much higher than scalp EEG,[2,49] the recognition of MEG normal variants is not trivial (**Figs. 10** and **11**).

The history of MEG is short compared with EEG, so the confidence in identifying normal physiologic variants is still maturing. Magnetoencephalographers are fortunate that they can build on their knowledge and experience with a variety of waveforms from EEG for the interpretation of MEG studies.[3] There are, however, the aforementioned normal variants that are ordinarily seen only in the MEG channels, and that will be unfamiliar to the novice magnetoencephalographer. Because the clinical application of MEG has its most critical role in the evaluation of patients with epilepsy in whom accurate localization of the epileptogenic zone is paramount for determination of their candidacy for resective surgery, distinguishing truly epileptic discharges from epileptiform-appearing variants is one of the most important tasks of the magnetoencephalographer.

SUMMARY AND FUTURE DIRECTIONS

Technological advancements have rapidly brought MEG from a research tool to a standard clinical test. As part of the standard of care in many centers, MEG is performed according to accepted

No definite EEG changes   Left parietal MEG sensors   Left posterior perisylvian benign variant

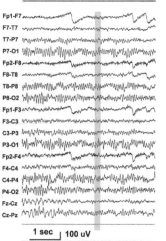

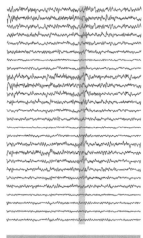

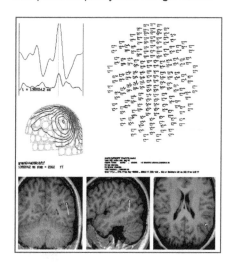

Fig. 10. Taken from an otherwise normal study, this figure illustrates one of the typical normal variants seen in MEG. The EEG, shown in a longitudinal bipolar montage shows no clear change. In the left parietal MEG sensors can be seen a relatively large transient, which has good dipolar pattern that localizes to the left posterior perisylvian region.

clinical practice guidelines.[10–12,50,51] The limitations in head coverage and spatial resolution have been eliminated by the progressive increase from the original 8 sensors, to 37, then to 128, and currently to whole head systems with 200 to 300 sensors. The technology needed to manufacture sensors has dramatically advanced, improving SNR and facilitating the recording of deep sources. Refilling the helium dewar used to be required once or twice per week, but helium recycling systems have greatly improved laboratory convenience and decreased operating costs. Tedious and complex digitization of HPI coils has been replaced by a variety of video, laser, and magnetic methods. Elimination of the requirement for patients to remain motionless during a MEG recording has opened up clinical MEG to a much wider range of pediatric and other patients who find it hard to cooperate.

In epilepsy, the analysis of resting state MEG, that is, without requiring any action of the patient and in the absence of interictal spikes, can provide an entirely new view of the malfunctioning operation of different brain regions, and promises to provide clinical results in those MEG cases that are otherwise considered negative.[52,53] There has been considerable research into the significance of high-frequency oscillations in the 80 to 500 Hz range, first measured with intracranial recording[54] and proposed as markers for the epileptogenic zone. High frequencies can be measured noninvasively by MEG[55,56] and MEG is being used to

record high-frequency oscillations for epilepsy localization.[57]

Applications beyond epilepsy and presurgical mapping have been the subject of considerable research efforts. These include autism, stroke, chronic pain, traumatic brain injury, Parkinson's disease, hepatic encephalopathy, neuropsychiatric disorders, dementia, and brain maturation.[58] Although not yet clinically applicable, MEG has been used to help identify biomarkers and track the progress of disease. MEG is especially useful for enhancing our understanding of brain connectivity, because its excellent time resolution lends itself to analysis of communication and propagation. The evaluation of brain connections may be carried out on spontaneous (ie, resting state) activity, or on activity that is evoked by some sort of stimulus (afferent or efferent). And of course, the MEG evaluation may investigate either normal interactions (such as regional synchronization between Wernicke's and Broca's areas during language processing, or connections between limbic and frontal cortex) or abnormal connections (such as between multiple suspected epileptogenic regions, or between the irritative zone and the seizure onset zone).

The cost and space requirements for MEG systems have limited the number of clinical MEG laboratories. Further hardware developments may eventually lead to sensors that can operate at room temperature. Systems using atomic magnetometry, also known as optically pumped

Right parietal MEG sensors

1 sec | 500 fT/cm

**Right central region
(Benign rolandic variant)**

**Colocalization with median
nerve SEF (shown in pink)**

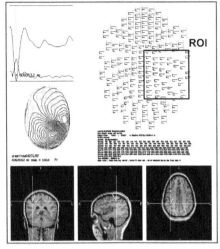

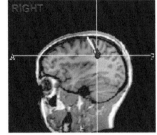

Fig. 11. This discharge in the right parietal MEG sensors was invisible on the simultaneously recorded EEG. In the middle panel, SECD source localization places this discharge in the posterior bank of the central sulcus. On the right, the typical co-localization of these benign rolandic discharges with the median nerve somatosensory evoked potential is shown.

magnetometry, which do not require liquid helium, are being developed.[59] The recent entry into the field of several new MEG hardware vendors will likely produce more advanced hardware and streamlined software, making MEG even more a part of the standard of care in epilepsy.

REFERENCES

1. Pataraia E, Simos PG, Castillo EM, et al. Does magnetoencephlography add to scalp video-EEG as a diagnostic tool in epilepsy surgery? Neurology 2004;62:943–8.
2. Stefan H, Hummel C, Scheler G, et al. Magnetic brain source imaging of focal epileptic activity: a synopsis of 455 cases. Brain 2003;126(11):2396–405.
3. Iwasaki M, Pestana E, Burgess RC, et al. Detection of epileptiform activity by human interpreters: blinded comparison between electroencephalography and magnetoencephalography. Epilepsia 2005;46(1):59–68.
4. Yoshinaga H, Nakahori T, Ohtsuka Y, et al. Benefit of simultaneous recording of EEG and MEG in dipole localization. Epilepsia 2002;43(8):924–8.
5. Oishi M, Otsubo H, Kameyama S, et al. Epileptic spikes: magnetoencephalography versus simultaneous electrocorticography. Epilepsia 2002;43:1390–5.
6. Cooper R, Winter AL, Crow HJ, et al. Comparison of subcortical, cortical, and scalp activity. Electroencephalogr Clin Neurophysiol 1965;18:217–28.
7. Tao JX, Ray A, Hawes-Ebersole S, et al. Intracranial EEG substrates. Epilepsia 2005;46(5):669–76.
8. Hamalainen M, Hari R, Ilmoneimi RJ. Magnetoencephalography—theory, instrumentation, and applications to noninvasive studies of the working brain. Rev Mod Phys 1993;65:413–97.
9. Hari R. Chapter 42. Magnetoencephalography: methods and applications. In: Shomer DL, Lopes da Silva FH, editors. Niedermeyer's Electroencephalography: Basic Principles, Clinical Applications, and Related Fields. 6th Edition. Philadelphia: Lippincott Williams & Wilkins; 2011. p. 865–900.
10. Bagic AI, Knowlton RC, Rose DF, et al. American Clinical Magnetoencephalography Society Clinical Practice Guideline 1: recording and analysis of spontaneous cerebral activity. J Clin Neurophysiol 2011;28(4):348–54.
11. Bagic AI, Knowleton RC, Rose DF, et al. American Clinical Magnetoencephlography Society Clinical Practice Guideline 3: MEG-EEG reporting. J Clin Neurophysiol 2011;28(4):362–3.
12. Bagic AI, Barkley GL, Rose DF, et al. American Clinical Magnetoencephalography Society Clinical Practice Guideline 4: qualifications of MEG-EEG personnel. J Clin Neurophysiol 2011;28(4):364–5.
13. Barkley GL, Baumgartner C. MEG and EEG in epilepsy. J Clin Neurophysiol 2003;20:163–78.
14. Kakisaka Y, Wang ZI, Mosher JC, et al. Clinical evidence for the utility of movement compensation algorithm in magnetoencephalography: successful localization during focal seizure. Epilepsy Res 2012;101(1–2):191–6.
15. Shibata S, Mosher JC, Kotagal P, et al. Magnetoencephalographic recordings in infants using a

standard- sized array: technical adequacy and diagnostic yield. J Clin Neurophysiol 2017;34(5): 461–8.

16. Lewine JD, Andrews R, Chez M, et al. Magnetoencephalographic patterns of epileptiform activity in children with regressive autism spectrum disorders. Pediatrics 1999;104:405–18.

17. Minassian BA, Otsubo H, Weiss S, et al. Magnetoencephalographic localization in pediatric epilepsy surgery: comparison with invasive intracranial electroencephalography. Ann Neurol 1999;46: 627–33.

18. Mohamed IS, Otsubo H, Ochi A, et al. Utility of magnetoencephalography in the evaluation of recurrent seizures after epilepsy surgery. Epilepsia 2007;48: 2150–9.

19. Otsubo H, Och A, Elliott I, et al. MEG predicts epileptic zone in lesional extrahippocampal epilepsy: 12 pediatric surgery cases. Epilepsia 2001; 42:1523–30.

20. Paetau R, Kajola M, Karhu J, et al. Magnetoencephalographic localization of epileptic cortex— impact on surgical treatment. Ann Neurol 1992;32: 106–9.

21. Paetau R, Hamalainen M, Hari R, et al. Magnetoencephalographic evaluation of children and adolescents with intractable epilepsy. Epilepsia 1994;35: 275–84.

22. Ramachandran Nair R, Otsubo H, Shroff MM, et al. MEG predicts outcome following surgery for intractable epilepsy in children with normal or nonfocal MRI findings. Epilepsia 2007;48:149–57.

23. Alkawadri R, Burgess RC, Kakisaka Y, et al. The utility of ictal magnetoencephalography in localization of seizure onset zone. JAMA Neurol 2018;75: 1264–72.

24. Almubarak S, Alexopoulos A, Von-Podewils F, et al. The correlation of magnetoencephalography to intracranial EEG in localizing the epileptogenic zone: a study of the surgical resection outcome. Epilepsy Res 2014;108:1581–90.

25. Shukla G, Kazutaka J, Gupta A, et al. Magnetoencephalographic identification of epileptic focus in children with generalized electroencephalographic (EEG) features but focal imaging abnormalities. J Child Neurol 2017;32(12):981–95.

26. Jerbi K, Mosher JC, Baillet S, et al. On MEG forward modelling using multipolar expansions. Phys Med Biol 2002;47(4):523–55.

27. Plummer C, Harvey AS, Cook M. EEG source localization in focal epilepsy: where are we now? Epilepsia 2008;49(2):201–18.

28. Ebersole JS, Ebersole SM. Combining MEG and EEG source modeling in epilepsy evaluations. J Clin Neurophysiol 2010;27(6):360–71.

29. Lantz G, Grave de Peralta R, Spinelli L, et al. Epileptic source localization with high density EEG:

how many electrodes are needed? Clin Neurophysiol 2003;114:63–9.

30. Eliashiv DS, Elsas SM, Squires K, et al. Ictal magnetic source imaging as a localizing tool in partial epilepsy. Neurology 2002;59:1600–10.

31. Iida K, Otsubo H, Mohamed IS, et al. Characterizing magnetoencephalographic spike sources in children with tuberous sclerosis complex. Epilepsia 2005;46(9):1510–7.

32. Mamelak AN, Lopez N, Akhtari M, et al. Magnetoencephalography-directed surgery in patients with neocortical epilepsy. J Neurosurg 2002;97(4): 865–73.

33. Ossenblok P, de Munck JC, Colon A, et al. Magnetoencephalography is more successful for screening and localizing frontal lobe epilepsy than electroencephalography. Epilepsia 2007;48:2139–49.

34. Bast T, Boppel T, Rupp A, et al. Noninvasive source localization of interictal EEG spikes: effects of signal- to-noise ratio and averaging. J Clin Neurophysiol 2006;23:487–97.

35. Bast T, Ramantani G, Boppel T, et al. Source analysis of interictal spikes in polymicrogyria: loss of relevant cortical fissures requires simultaneous EEG to avoid MEG misinterpretation. Neuroimage 2005;25(4):1232–41.

36. Wennberg R, Cheyne D. Reliability of MEG source imaging of anterior temporal spikes: analysis of an intracranially characterized spike focus. Clin Neurophysiol 2014;125:903–18.

37. Genow A, Hummel C, Scheler G, et al. Epilepsy surgery, resection volume and MSI localization in lesional frontal lobe epilepsy. NeuroImage 2004;21: 444–9.

38. Scheler G, Fischer MJM, Genow A, et al. Spatial relationship of source localizations in patients with focal epilepsy: comparison of MEG and EEG with a three spherical shells and a boundary element volume conductor model. Hum Brain Mapp 2007;28: 315–22.

39. Mosher JC, Spencer ME, Leahy RM, et al. Error bounds for EEG and MEG dipole source localization. Electroencephalogr Clin Neurophysiol 1993; 86:303–21.

40. Gavaret M, Badier JM, Bartolomei F, et al. MEG and EEG sensitivity in a case of medial occipital epilepsy. Brain Topogr 2014;27(1):192–6.

41. Leahy RM, Mosher JC, Spencer ME, et al. A study of dipole localization accuracy for MEG and EEG using a human skull phantom. Electroencephalogr Clin Neurophysiol 1998;107:159–73.

42. Janszky J, Jokeit H, Schulz R, et al. EEG predicts surgical outcome in lesional frontal lobe epilepsy. Neurology 2000;54:1470–6.

43. Baillet S, Mosher S, Leahy RM. Electromagnetic brain mapping. IEEE Signal Process Mag 2001; 18(6):14–30.

44. Hillebrand A, Barnes GR. A quantitative assessment of the sensitivity of whole-head MEG to activity in the adult human cortex. NeuroImage 2002;16(3):638–50.

45. Vadera S, Jehi L, Burgess RC, et al. Correlation between magnetoencephalography-based "clusterectomy" and postoperative seizure freedom. Neurosurg Focus 2013;34(6):E9 (1–4).

46. Murakami H, Wang ZI, Marashly A, et al. Correlating magnetoencephalography to stereo- electroencephalography in patients undergoing epilepsy surgery. Brain 2016;135(11):2935–47.

47. Taulu S, Simola J. Spatiotemporal signal space separation method for rejecting nearby interference in MEG measurements. Phys Med Biol 2006;51(7):1759–68.

48. Benbadis SR. Just like EKGs! Should EEGs undergo a confirmatory interpretation by a clinical neurophysiologist? Neurology 2013;80(Suppl. 1):S47–51.

49. Knake S, Halgren E, Shiraishi H, et al. The value of multichannel MEG and EEG in the presurgical evaluation of 70 epilepsy patients. Epilepsy Res 2006;69:80–6.

50. Burgess RC, Barkley GL, Bagic AI. Turning a new page in clinical magnetoencephalography: practicing according to the first clinical practice guidelines. J Clin Neurophysiol 2011;28(4):339–40.

51. Burgess RC, Funke ME, Bowyer SM, et al. American Clinical Magnetoencephalography Society Clinical Practice Guideline 2: presurgical functional brain mapping using magnetic evoked fields. J Clin Neurophysiol 2011;28(4):355–61.

52. Elisevich K, Shukla N, Moran JE, et al. An assessment of MEG coherence imaging in the study of temporal lobe epilepsy. Epilepsia 2011;52(6):1110–9.

53. Krishnan B, Vlachos I, Wang ZI, et al. Epileptic focus localization based on resting state interictal MEG recordings is feasible irrespective of the presence or absence of spikes. Clin Neurophysiol 2015;126(4):667–74.

54. Bragin A, Engel J, Wilson CL, et al. High-frequency oscillations in human brain. Hippocampus 1999;9:37–142.

55. Muthukumaraswamy SD, Singh KD. Visual gamma oscillations: the effects of stimulus type, visual field coverage and stimulus motion on MEG and EEG recordings. NeuroImage 2013;69:223–30.

56. Rampp S, Kaltenhauser M, Weigel D, et al. MEG correlates of epileptic high gamma oscillations in invasive EEG. Epilepsia 2010;51(8):1638–42.

57. Heers M, Jacobs J, Hirschmann J, et al. Spike associated high frequency oscillations in magnetoencephalography co-localize with focal cortical dysplasia type IIB. Epilepsia 2013;54(Suppl. 3):4–21.

58. Hari R, Baillet S, Barnes G, et al. IFCN-endorsed practical guidelines for clinical magnetoencephalography (MEG). Clin Neurophysiol 2018;129(8):1720–47.

59. Boto E, Holmes N, Leggett J, et al. Moving magnetoencephalography towards real-world applications with a wearable system. Nature 2018;555:657–61.

Presurgical Functional Mapping with Magnetoencephalography

Susan M. Bowyer, PhD[a],*, Elizabeth W. Pang, PhD[b],
Mingxiong Huang, PhD[c], Andrew C. Papanicolaou, PhD[d],
Roland R. Lee, MD[c]

KEYWORDS

- Magnetoencephalography • Presurgical • Mapping • Somatosensory evoked magnetic fields
- Motor evoked magnetic fields • Auditory evoked magnetic fields • Visual evoked magnetic fields
- Language evoked magnetic fields

KEY POINTS

- Magnetoencephalography (MEG) can noninvasively localize the primary somatosensory cortex.
- MEG can noninvasively localize the primary motor cortex.
- MEG can noninvasively localize the primary auditory cortex.
- MEG can noninvasively localize the primary visual cortex.
- MEG can noninvasively localize the language areas.

INTRODUCTION

Localization of the eloquent cortex, prior to a surgical resection, is vital to ensure a good outcome for a patient's quality of life. Noninvasive magneto-encephalography (MEG) imaging can provide presurgical mapping of functional locations and networks in the brain. Brain disorders, such as epilepsy and tumors, can have an effect on the location of the primary sensory, motor, auditory, visual, and language processing areas because they often undergo functional reorganization if these areas of the brain are invaded by a tumor or epileptogenic tissue. Tumors and epileptic tissue may also cause changes in the neuronal networks subserving these various functions, which can result in decreased MEG-signal amplitude, increased latency, or importantly, change in location of eloquent cortex. These changes, if they have occurred, must be located before surgery in order to plan a surgical resection that will maximize preservation of eloquent cortex, while still effecting a complete resection of the tumor or epileptic tissue, thus preserving a good quality of life following surgery.

Many MEG studies have investigated the process of mapping the locations of the cortical areas containing parts of neuronal cortex supporting somatosensory, motor, auditory, visual, and language functions. In this article, the authors review how these MEG studies and MEG protocols can be used for presurgical functional mapping.

Functional Localization: the Method

The finished MEG result, which displays the MEG source localization onto the patient's magnetic resonance (MR) image, is called magnetic source imaging (MSI) and involves obtaining a good-quality volumetric MR imaging that is used to

[a] MEG Lab, Henry Ford Hospital, Wayne State University, CFP 079, 2799 West Grand Boulevard, Detroit, MI 48202, USA; [b] Division of Neurology, Hospital for Sick Children, University of Toronto, 555 University Avenue, Toronto, Ontario M5G 1X8, Canada; [c] UCSD Radiology Imaging Laboratory, University of California San Diego, VA San Diego Healthcare System, 3510 Dunhill Street, San Diego, CA 92121, USA; [d] The University of Tennessee, College of Medicine, 910 Madison Avenue # 1002, Memphis, TN 38103, USA
* Corresponding author.
E-mail address: sbowyer1@hfhs.org

Neuroimag Clin N Am 30 (2020) 159–174
https://doi.org/10.1016/j.nic.2020.02.005

coregister to the MEG source space that was recorded by the head position coils (3–5 coils are needed) during the MEG recording. Recording magnetic fields at the head surface requires an extremely sensitive recording device (a superconducting quantum interference device) and sophisticated software programs. The magnetic fields can be recorded with recording systems consisting of 100 to 350 sensors or coils, using either magnetometers, planar gradiometers, or axial gradiometers. A study by Bardouille and colleagues[1] showed that the S1 median nerve sensory localization is not biased by the type of MEG system coil used. For functional mapping, the magnetic fields around the head are recorded for 5 to 10 minutes while a stimulus is applied to the sensory area of interest. The stimulus for the main 5 evoked field mappings typically includes the following:

- Tapping of the fingers or electrical stimulation of the median nerve for sensory stimulation
- Moving of the finger to press a button or move an accelerometer for motor stimulation
- Listening to tones presented at 500 or 1000 Hz for auditory stimulation
- Visually looking at a reversing black-and-white checkerboard pattern at 1 Hz for visual stimulation
- Listening to words, or looking at written words or pictures, for language stimulation

While recording the MEG data, a trigger must be included that indicates the latency at which the stimulation was applied; this allows for the data to be segmented into epochs and then averaged together. Trying to look at a single stimulation trial is difficult, because the brain signal may be very close to the background noise level of the brain. Therefore, by averaging 50 or more trials of the stimulation events together, the brain signal can be boosted enough that it can be clearly seen above the background brain activity. The authors review how many trials are needed to create a good response that can be used to clearly localize the evoked magnetic field response for each type of stimulation.

The MEG source localization procedure can be performed using several different types of software programs, ranging from commercially available platforms (Curry, ASA, BESA, ESME) to packages developed in different laboratories to answer specific clinical and/or research questions. These software programs are, in many cases, open-source toolboxes (eg, Brainstorm, EEGlab, FieldTrip, MEG-TOOLS, MNE, NutMEG, Open-MEEG, Simbio, SPM, VBMEG, MEG Processor). These programs use different types of source

localization approaches, such as single equivalent current dipole (ECD), multidipole, minimum norm, or beamformer approaches. Presurgical mapping of the primary sensory, motor, auditory, and visual cortex has been performed mainly with the ECD technique and so have many language mapping studies. However, where appropriate, additional techniques may provide complementary information. When the ECD model is used, it is desirable to use only those channels that contain the isofield map for dipole fitting (see, eg, Ref.[2]).

To ensure good-quality MEG recording from all types of evoked magnetic field responses, the patient should be awake and cooperative. Therefore, adequate sleep of the patient before any testing is essential. Because the epilepsy mapping sessions are usually performed when the patient is sleep deprived, some laboratories require the patient to return for somatosensory and language mapping on a different day. All procedures ought to be repeated for the purpose of establishing test-retest reliability. A recent study looking at repeated MEG localizations of the median nerve stimulation (S1) over 3 different days found the variability of the 35 milliseconds (N30m) peak location in each subject was 4.9 ± 1.9 mm per session and 8.3 ± 3.4 mm per day.[3]

Inspection of the raw data is mandatory in order to allow identification and discarding of noise-contaminated trials or suboptimally performing channels. It is preferable to record continuous MEG data and simultaneously record triggers on another channel for ease of dividing the data into segments and averaging them. Advanced MEG data analysis of the network activity using coherence and connectivity analysis is also facilitated with the use of continuous data instead of epoch data.

METHODS OF ACQUISITION AND ANALYSIS OF EVOKED MAGNETIC FIELDS
Somatosensory Evoked Magnetic Fields

MEG has sufficient spatial resolution to reveal the organization of primary somatosensory cortex with a very high success rate,[4] using either mechanical stimulation of the fingertips, toes, and lip corner[5–7] or electrical stimulation of the median and tibial nerves.[4,8] The sources of the early- and middle-latency components of magnetic responses (occurring <60 milliseconds after stimulus onset) and modeled as successive single ECDs, originate in the contralateral primary sensory cortex. The postcentral gyrus includes the primary somatosensory cortex (Brodmann areas 3, 2, and 1) collectively referred to as S1. In general, somatosensory stimuli evoke early cortical components

(N25, P30, P60, N80) generated in the contralateral primary somatosensory cortex (S1), related to the processing of the physical stimulus attributes. The N20 peak is usually detected under the C4-P4 electrodes, whereas the P60 is detected under Cz in the electroencephalogram (EEG) recordings. To differentiate the MEG response from the EEG response, the "m" is added so the N20 EEG response becomes the N20m MEG response (N25, N25m; P60, P60m, N80, N80m). The MEG coil array geometry will determine if the largest evoked peak is detected directly under the coil, as would be the case with a planar gradiometer coil, or off to the side where the maximum magnetic field was exiting the head, as would be the case in a magnetometer or axial gradiometer coil system.

The efficacy of MEG for somatosensory mapping has been established in large-scale studies with patients sustaining space-occupying lesions[5] (see also Ref.[4]). The accuracy of MEG for presurgical cortical mapping has been established in the primary somatosensory cortex (S1) via comparison to invasive mapping, which is the gold-standard mapping method,[9] and by surgical outcome.[5,10] MEG was found to be superior to functional magnetic resonance (fMR) imaging for locating the central sulcus, because activation of multiple nonprimary cerebral areas may confound the interpretation of functional MR imaging results.[8]

Indications for somatosensory evoked magnetic fields (SEF) mapping include abnormal sensations associated with the onset of seizures, or associated with tumor, especially tumors in the vicinity of the postcentral gyrus.

Somatosensory evoked magnetic field in the pediatric population

The recording of the somatosensory evoked potential in children for epilepsy surgery and presurgical mapping for brain tumors is also well established.[4,11,12] The SEF can be recorded in infants[13] and in children with parameters comparable to those used in adults.[14,15] SEFs can be acquired with sedation in children.[16]

Somatosensory evoked magnetic field stimulation

Sites of electrical stimulation frequently used in clinical SEF examination include the median nerve and tibial nerve. Mechanical stimuli can be used for fingers, lips, tongue, and other regions of the body.

Mechanical stimulation Mechanical stimulation devices producing air puffs or taps may be used. Tactile stimulation may not produce results that are as reliable as electrical stimulation, but there are well-established routines for using this type of stimulation. Mechanical stimulation is easier to use and better tolerated in infants and toddlers. Stimulation taps are rapidly applied to a single digit. Stimulators can also be attached to the lip or the toes.

Electrical stimulation Stimulus amplitude should be adjusted for individual patients so that the motor threshold is excited to cause a clearly visible twitch of the thumb. Typical stimulus amplitudes required for achieving a twitch range from 5 to 10 mA. The stimulating electrode impedance should be 5 kΩ or less. The aggregate stimulus frequency should be less than 5 Hz even if distributed to multiple stimulation sites. Electrode placements for stimulation of the median nerve should be on the wrist, spaced about 1 inch apart.

Somatosensory evoked magnetic field recording parameters

Data acquisition parameters for electrical stimulation A bandpass of 0.03 to 300 Hz with a digitization rate of 1000 Hz is preferred but could be 0.01 to 100 Hz, digitized at 508 Hz. Real-time averaging is useful in determining the number of necessary trials for achieving sufficient SNR. Two hundred to 500 trials are typically required to yield adequate average responses. Averaging off-line following data collection permits the application of noise-reduction routines and manual or automatic artifact rejection. Epoch duration of 250 milliseconds with an additional 50 milliseconds prestimulus baseline and an interstimulus interval (ISI) of 500 to 2000 milliseconds are typically used.

Data acquisition for mechanical stimulation A bandpass of 0.1 to 100 Hz with a digitization rate of 508.63 Hz is typically used. 512 trials yield an adequate number of acceptable trials. Epochs of 400 milliseconds in duration, 100 milliseconds prestimulus baseline, and an ISI of 600 milliseconds are recommended.

Somatosensory evoked magnetic field localization

Before analysis of the localization of the N30m and P40m, the data need to be filtered correctly to view these peaks. If the data are filtered 0.5 to 50 Hz or wider, and there is low-frequency noise, the N30m response will not be seen. The data must be filtered 8 to 40 Hz, as seen in **Fig. 1**. The 2 peaks become clearer with this finer filter setting. Depending on the software used, the MEG and MR imaging source spaces will need to be coregistered, and this will provide the anatomic background for the MEG sources.

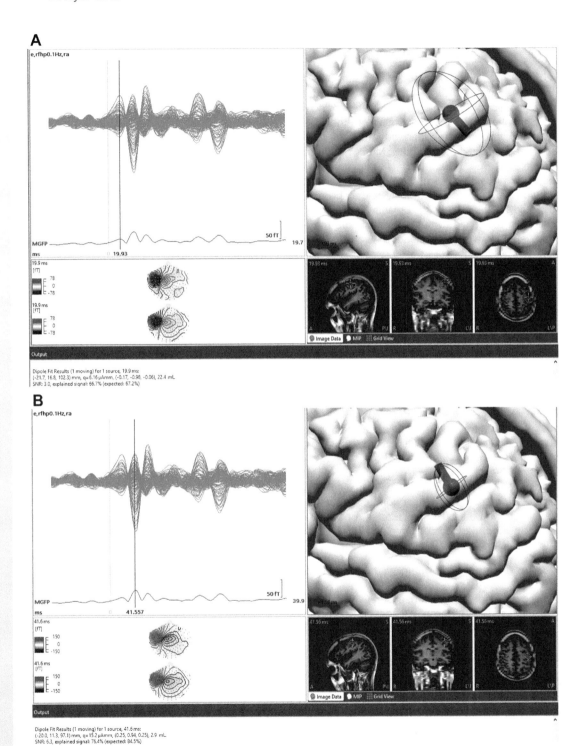

Fig. 1. A 26-year-old right-handed female with intractable localization related epilepsy had her SEF response mapped during mechanical tapping of the index finger. Curry software using all 148 channels of MEG magnetometers to localize (*A*) N30m response seen at 20 milliseconds, and (*B*) P40m response seen at 41 milliseconds. Note the dipole is located in the left postcentral gyrus, and the orientation of the dipole is 180° different between the latencies (Subject ID MN 20252).

After the data are filtered 8 to 40 Hz, the peak near the 30-milliseconds latency is selected, and dipole-fit algorithm is performed to determine where in the cortex the best estimate for this source is. For the ECD, a dot with a tail will be located on the posterior bank of the central sulcus. The direction of the tip and the tail will denote the direction of the intercellular current flow. The model indicates the current flows from the tip to the tail. In the cortex, the dendrites are all lined up perpendicular to the cortical surface. The current flows from the surface of the cortex to the interior of the cortex. This orientation of the current flow and how the dipole is modeled allow one to check if the dipole is on the correct bank of a sulcus.

SEF maps are acquired as a standard procedure at many MEG center locations. The SEF is very useful for identifying where the central sulcus is located as well as determining if the SEF has undergone any functional reorganization because of a tumor or epileptogenic tissue.

Movement-Related Evoked Magnetic Fields

Several activation protocols for the identification of the motor cortex have been developed.[9,17] Movement-related evoked magnetic fields (MEFs) arise from a readiness potential that precedes a finger or body moment by 1 to 5 seconds, and this potential is widely distributed over the motor-related areas in both hemispheres.[18] Many MEG studies have investigated the MEF response in the precentral gyrus that can be detected by MEG 40 to 60 milliseconds before movement.[18–22] There are several areas in the cortex that are activated during movement. These areas include the primary motor cortex, also called M1, and several premotor areas, such as the supplementary motor area (SMA), pre-supplementary motor area (pre-SMA), and ventral and dorsal parts of the premotor cortex (PMC).

MEG studies using a finger button-press procedure have been successful in providing data of adequate quality for clinical use.[4] In some studies, the sources of MEFs preceding EMG onset by approximately 50 to 100 milliseconds have been modeled as single, successive ECDs.[8,10] In other studies, sources have been estimated using spatial filtering algorithms, such as beamformers.[4]

The Fast-VESTAL spatiotemporal L1-minimum norm algorithm,[23] described in Matti Hämäläinen and colleagues' article, "MEG Signal Processing, Forward Modeling, MEG Inverse Source Imaging, and Coherence Analysis," in this issue, can routinely localize the primary motor cortex of hands, face, or ankle movement. The precentral gyrus includes the primary motor cortex (Brodmann area 4).

The primary indications for MEF mapping include the proximity of the lesion to be resected to the primary motor cortex. MEG's good temporal resolution also allows the detection of abnormal latency in MEF due to brain tumors. Brain tumors can cause a significant delay in the MEF, and decreased signal amplitude.[24]

Movement-related evoked magnetic fields in the pediatric population
Motor evoked fields cannot be acquired in infants or sedated children, but can be acquired in cooperative children as young as 4 years of age.[25,26] The parameters used with adults may be used with children.

Movement-related evoked magnetic fields stimulation
Motor stimulation is activated during finger tapping that is self-paced or cued (visually or auditorily). This task is very tiring to have a patient perform. The timing of the tapping can be recorded by pressing a button or isometric contractions that interrupt a light beam. Somatosensory cue-initiated simultaneous recording of somatosensory and motor responses can be performed[10], where tactile stimulation activates initially the contralateral primary somatosensory cortex followed by activation of the secondary somatosensory cortex, lasting for approximately 150 ms. Activity in the contralateral precentral gyrus is seen next immediately preceding the onset of electromyographic activity marking the onset of finger movement. Finally, somatosensory activity is again observed during the movement, presumably the result of proprioceptive input.[10]

Movement-related evoked magnetic fields recording parameters
The bandpass is typically set at 0.1 to 100 Hz, and the digitization rate is typically set at 508.63 Hz. Continuous MEG data acquisition is best during the performance of 50 to 100 finger tappings. Epochs will be averaged based on the trigger from visual or auditory cue or from a button press. In the case of the simultaneous SEF and MEF recordings, the tactile stimulus from the SEF can be used as the averaging trigger. Epoch durations depend on the intermovement interval (IMI). Epochs of 3-second duration would include a 500-millisecond baseline and 200 milliseconds after the trigger recording, along with the IMI of about 1 to 2 seconds.

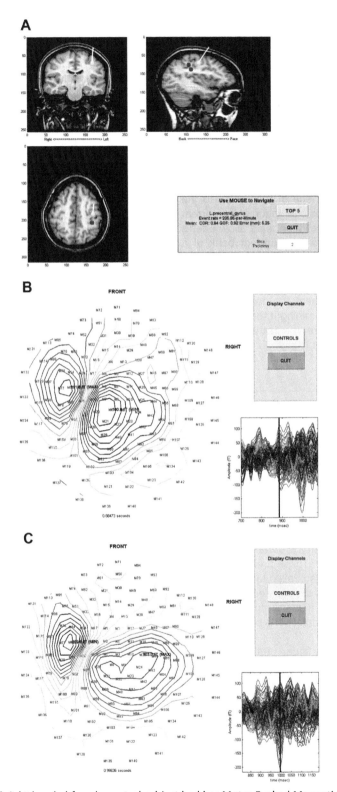

Fig. 2. A 43-year-old right-handed female control subject had her Motor Evoked Magnetic Fields (MEF) mapped by pressing a button after an auditory cue. (*A*) The motor response (MEF) in the precentral gyrus (*yellow*) preceded the sensory response (SEF) in the post central gyrus (*red*) from pushing a response pad button. (*B*) Displays the magnetic contour plot of the MEF at 884ms after an auditory cue to press the button followed by (*C*) the SEF response to the button press at 996ms. Note the MEF and SEF response is not very robust. (Subject ID 5514i).

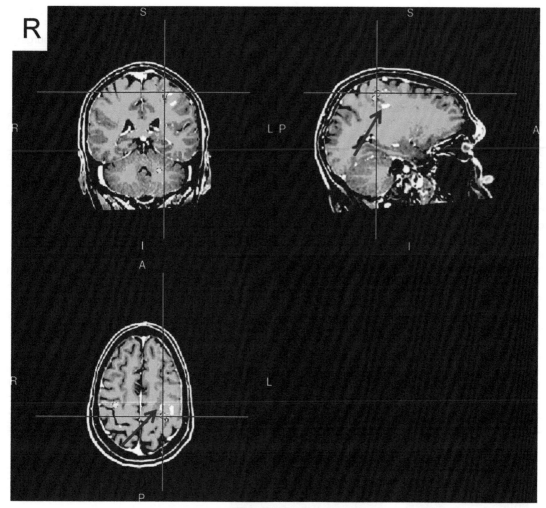

Fig. 3. A 52-year-old man with left frontal lobe melanoma metastasis. Right-hand primary motor cortex is localized by the Fast-VESTAL algorithm, using a repeating hand-clench paradigm for 2 minutes of data acquisition preceded by 15 seconds of baseline resting state. The enhancing tumor is marked by the pink arrow. The source activation map shows the right-hand motor cortex (*yellow patch* and *crosshairs*) is located just posterior to the posterior left frontal lobe enhancing mass. The contralateral left-hand motor cortex is also shown on the axial image and localizes as expected to the anterior bank of right central sulcus.

Movement-related evoked magnetic fields localization

Prior to analysis of the localization of the motor responses, the data need to have 50 to 100 events averaged together after they had been inspected to have artifacts removed. The data should be filtered 8 to 40 Hz. Inspection of the waveform for a peak 80 to 100 milliseconds before the SEF should be seen and selected for the dipole fit algorithm to be performed. The ECD fit will determine where in the cortex the best estimate for this sources is. **Fig. 2** displays the MEG dipole locations of the MEF. The patient in **Fig. 2** moved their right index finger to an auditory cue 50 times. The MEF is located in the precentral gyrus (yellow). The red

dots indicate the SEF that was also recorded as the finger touched the button. The SEF is on the opposite bank of the central sulcus in the postcentral gyrus. The current flow from the surface of the cortex to the interior of the cortex allows one to determine if the dipole is located on the correct bank of the sulcus. The magnetic field contour maps and the 148 channels of averaged MEG data are displayed; the line in the waveform indicates the MEF (884 ms) and the SEF (996 ms) approximately 112ms apart.

MEF maps are not usually acquired at some MEG center locations. The MEF can be a difficult field to identify in the MEG data. This task is also tiring for the patient, and robust MEG data are not usually collected. However, using the Fast-VESTAL analysis[23] as described above, standard data acquisitions routinely provide accurate localization of the motor cortex (Fig. 3).

Auditory Evoked Magnetic Fields

Auditory functioning can be determined by detecting the activation of the N100 response to sounds. MEG is a robust method to measure the latency and location of the N100m auditory response.[27-29] Auditory information is processed by the brain in the contralateral, superior part of the temporal lobe to the ear that hears the stimulus. The superior temporal gyrus includes the primary auditory cortex (Brodmann areas 41 and 42) and is often referred to as Heschl gyrus. The auditory cortex is arranged tonotopically, meaning that as the frequency heard increases, then the location on the cortex that receives this information moves into the deeper regions of the brain (medially).[30,31] Therefore, a 500-Hz tone would localize more laterally on the auditory cortex than a 5000-Hz tone would. In general, auditory stimulation will evoke a cortical component approximately 100 milliseconds after the tone is presented in the contralateral primary auditory cortex. This response is called the auditory N100 or N100m in MEG. The earlier components in the brainstem are not well recorded by MEG.

Significant delay in the latency of the auditory N100m component was detected by AEF in patients with temporal lobe tumor, and after surgery, the abnormally prolonged N100m latency returned to the normal range.[32] The signal amplitude was also lower in the abnormal compared to the normal side.

Localization of the primary auditory cortex is useful for planning lesion resections that encroach on the superior temporal plane.[32,33]

Indications for auditory evoked magnetic fields (AEF) mapping include abnormal hearing sensation associated with the onset of seizures, or associated with tumors, especially tumors in the vicinity of the auditory cortex.

Auditory evoked magnetic fields in the pediatric population

AEFs have been studied sufficiently in children and can be reliably acquired using the same parameters as in adults, although in young children, a longer ISI is recommended,[34,35] and very long ISIs are preferred for infants.[36]

Auditory evoked magnetic fields stimulation

In many cases AEF can be obtained by monaural or binaural stimulation of a pure tone that is well heard. Usually a 1000-Hz tone is presented monaurally, through headphones, unless tonotopic mapping is called for, in which case tones

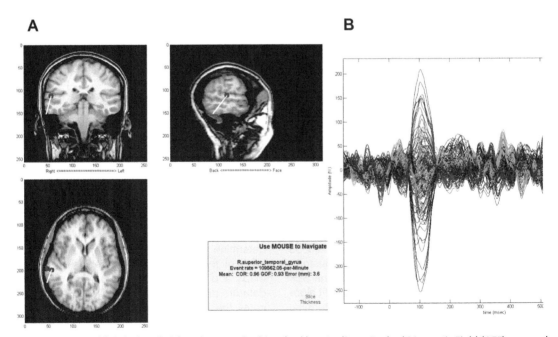

Fig. 4. A 39-year-old right-handed female control subject had her Auditory Evoked Magnetic Field (AEF) mapped by listening to a 500Hz tone presented in the left ear. (*A*) 37 channels of MEG magnetometers were used to localize the N100m response in the right superior temporal gyrus. (*B*) Display of all 148 MEG channel averaged waveform illustrates the robust auditory magnetic field response at 94ms. (Subject ID 5514d).

of different frequencies would be used. The intensity of the stimuli is usually 60 dB above hearing threshold for 50- to 200-milliseconds duration, and an ISI of 1second is frequently used.

Auditory evoked magnetic fields recoding parameters

The bandpass is usually set at 0.1 to 100 Hz, and a digitization rate of 508.63 Hz is adequate for this purpose. A minimum of 100 to 200 trials may be required to yield an adequate number of acceptable trials for the computation of a clear AEF.

Auditory evoked magnetic fields localization

Prior to analysis of the localization of the N100m, the data need to be averaged together and filtered. Using a tight bandpass filter of 1 to 30 Hz will provide a wide enough window to clearly see the N100m AEF response. **Fig. 4** shows the MEG dipole and the MEG data from all 148 MEG channels. The waveform display is in a butterfly plot of the MEG channels where the strong N100m AEF response can be seen at 94ms after the tone was presented. The AEF response was evoked by listening to 100 repeated tones at 500 Hz, presented monaurally to the left ear. Only 37 channels of MEG magnetometers over the right temporal lobe were used to localize the N100m response.

AEF maps are acquired as a standard at many MEG center locations. The AEF is very useful for identifying if there are any problems with hearing, or determining if the AEF has undergone any functional reorganization owing to a tumor or epileptogenic tissue.

Visual Evoked Magnetic Fields

MEG mapping of the primary visual processing has been performed for many years with MEG.[37,38] Primary visual processing (V1) occurs in the occipital cortex (Brodmann area 17). There are 3 distinct waveforms that can be evoked during a change in light pattern perceived by the contralateral eye. The N75m, P100m, and N145m provide information on visual pathway dysfunctions. Hemifield or single-quadrant stimulation has been successfully used to localize the visual cortex in patients before surgical interventions.[5,39,40] Mapping the visual pathways and the precise location of the primary visual cortex may be required to successfully remove a tumor and leave visual processing intact.[41–44]

Indication for visual evoked magnetic fields (VEF) is abnormal vision associated with the onset of seizure, or associated with tumor or lesion. VEF mapping is used to localize the primary visual cortex and its spatial relation to epileptiform activity sources and/or lesions.

Visual evoked magnetic fields in the pediatric population

There are no adaptations necessary to record VEF in children. The parameters used in the adult population are identical to those used with children. The basic VEF to a checkerboard reversal has been studied in typically developing children.[45]

Visual evoked magnetic fields stimulation

VEF are typically recorded in response to an alternating (1 Hz) checkerboard pattern. The size of the checkerboard is important, as the smaller the checkerboard the longer the latency and the smaller the amplitude of the VEF response.[43] Check sizes of approximately 30' to 60' of visual arc are best. This pattern is viewed on a projection screen in front of the patient. Patients are asked to lay or sit still, keeping their eyes open and focused on a colored dot in the center of their field of view.

Visual evoked magnetic fields recording parameters

VEF are usually recorded with the bandpass set between 0.1 and 100 Hz and sampled at 508 Hz. One hundred to 500 trials are typically needed for the pattern reversal to provide a sufficiently clear average signal. Each epoch contains 1 cycle of a black-and-white alternating checkerboard pattern flash. Real-time averaging is optional and may help to determine the number of necessary trials for computing a clear average waveform. Hemifields are recorded when only half of the checkerboard pattern reverses, whereas quarterfields are recorded when only a quarter of the checkerboard pattern is reversing. These hemi and quarter field stimulations provide for a more precise mapping of the visual cortex.

Visual evoked magnetic fields localization

Prior to analysis of the localization of the visual responses, the data need to have the 100 to 500 events averaged together after they had been inspected to have artifacts removed. The data should be filtered 8 to 40 Hz. Inspection of the waveform for a peak 70 to 150 milliseconds after the visual pattern reverses will be selected for the dipole fit algorithm. The ECD fit will determine where in the cortex the best estimate for these sources for the N75m, P100m, and N145m visual responses are located. **Fig. 5** displays the MEG dipole locations of the VEF.

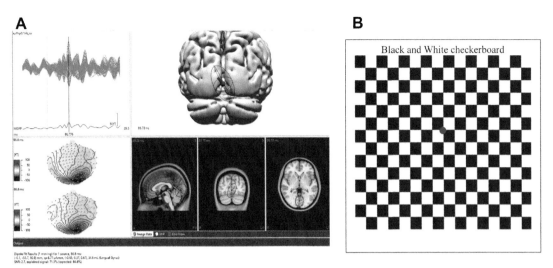

Fig. 5. A 21-year-old right-handed male control subject had his Visual Evoked Magnetic Field (VEF) mapped during a right visual hemi field stimulation. The subject focused on the red dot in the center of the black-and-white checkerboard pattern, and only the right half of the checkerboard is reversed at 1 Hz (1 per second) seen in (B). Responses are collected for each eye separately during 100 pattern reversals. Curry software using all 148 channels of MEG magnetometers was used to localize the P100m field. (A) During the right-eye stimulation the P100m, response is seen at 87 milliseconds; the N75m peak can be seen at 67 milliseconds, and the N145m peak can be seen at 122 milliseconds. Note the dipole for the P100m response is located in the left calcarine fissure for stimulation of the right visual field. The orientation of the dipole is such that the current flows from the tip to the tail, also indicating the bank of the gyral surface in the left hemisphere. The dipole fit parameters are listed below the figure and indicate that 71% of the signal is explained by this dipole mode, and the volume of the red ellipsoid is 34.6 mL, indicating that the confidence is within this region (Subject ID 5500).

VEF maps are easily acquired at most MEG center locations. The P100m VEF response is easily identified in the MEG data, and its latency and location can be used to determine if the VEF has undergone any functional reorganization because of a tumor or epileptogenic tissue.

Language-Related Evoked Magnetic Fields

Recording of language-related evoked magnetic fields (LEFs) has 2 main clinical indications: First, to establish the profile of hemispheric dominance for language and second, to identify the location and extent of functionally intact cortex involved in language functions. The determination of the hemisphere that is dominant for language is based on the accurate localization of Broca's and Wernicke's activated areas during language processing. Several tasks ranging from semantic decision making, verb generation, picture naming, to auditory word presentation have been used with success.[46–48] In general, most right-handed individuals are left-hemispheric dominant for language. Therefore, indication for mapping the LEFs is abnormal speech or language processing associated with the onset of seizure, or associated with tumor or lesion. If there is a lesion/tumor or

epileptic tissue that is in or near the location of the language processing areas, then identification of how the functional tissue has reorganized in relation to the area to be resected needs to be identified. LEF localizations will provide information on deficits the patient may experience after surgery is complete.

Lateralization of Language Function

The dominant hemisphere for language is based on an assessment of how much language activity is evoked in each hemisphere. Laterality indices can be calculated from the number of ECD dipoles found in each hemisphere, with the highest value being considered the language-dominant hemisphere. Amplitude of the current occurring in each hemisphere can be used to determine laterality, with the highest value being considered the language-dominant hemisphere. Several laboratories have verified that MEG assessments of hemispheric dominance for language are concordant with those based on the Wada or intracarotid amobarbital procedure (IAP) results approximately 93% of the time.[46,48–59] There are several activation protocols for eliciting brain responses to linguistic material that are detailed below under receptive (incoming stimuli) to expressive (output speech). Concordance rates between independent clinical judgments based on MEG and on the Wada procedure range from 87% and higher. Equally high are the sensitivity and the specificity.[52,60] Comparable concordance rates have been obtained between the results of invasive methods and MEG using a variety of activation tasks and extended-source modeling techniques.[54,56,58,59] Finally, a concordance rate over 90% has been reported using another extended-source modeling algorithm (MR-FOCUSS) in the context of a verbal generation and a naming task.[48]

Procedures for Assessing Hemispheric Dominance for Receptive Language

Receptive area of language function is the ability to understand words (i.e., supporting linguistic processing of the meaning of the word). This receptive area on the cortex is in the posterior part of the superior temporal gyrus (STG), which is also known as Wernicke's area and/or Brodmann's Area (BA) 22. The supramarginal gyrus (BA40) and the angular gyrus (BA39) are extended areas involved in phonological and articulatory processing (SMG) of words as well as semantic processing (ANG). These are areas that can be activated during auditory and/or visual processing of language.[61,62] The MEG studies that were previously validated with the Wada or IAP test used a receptive language task where the patient passively listened to auditory words or passively read visually presented words.[46,48-59]

The accuracy of these LEF cortical estimates has been verified against the results of invasive intra- or extraoperative electrocortical stimulation mapping (ECS).[63] Specifically, electrical stimulation of the cortical surface corresponding to these ECD clusters reliably impaired repetition of aurally presented sentences. More recently, spatial filtering was used to localize receptive-language related brain activity in 47 patients who later underwent ECS.[64] A total of 63 language-specific cortical sites were identified by MEG, of which 55 sites (87%) were verified using ECS (within ~ 1cm). Verification between MEG and ECS were based most commonly on repetition errors (78%), followed by naming errors (37%).

Procedures for Assessing Hemispheric Dominance for Expressive Language

Expressive areas of the brain are activated during motor speech (when language is expressed, just prior to mouth movement during spoken speech).[65] This speech processing language area is known as Broca's area. Broca's area is a cortical region in the inferior frontal lobe, also known as BA 45: pars triangularis and BA 44: pars opercularis. To activate expressive language processing and Broca's area supporting motor speech, subjects should be instructed to engage in an expressive task, such as covertly naming images or silently generating verbs. MEG studies have been performed to assess hemispheric dominance for expressive language. Kober and colleagues[66] reported success in eliciting inferior frontal activity using a picture-naming task and a spatial filtering algorithm to model cortical sources of neuromagnetic activity. Hirata and colleagues[57] also used spatial filtering to model activity in the beta band recorded during performance of a silent word-reading task in 12 patients with epilepsy or tumors. They reported an average distance of 6.0 ± 7.1 mm between the intraoperative stimulation site(s) associated with speech arrest and the cortical patches that displayed significant activation in the inferior or middle frontal gyri. Bowyer and colleagues[53] successfully used an object-naming task to localize activity in Broca's area. This study used a current distribution technique (MR-FOCUSS)[67] to localize activity in the left inferior frontal gyrus (IFG) area. The latency for this activity was seen at 436 +/- 40 ms across all subjects.[53] Similarly, the distributed source L1-minimum norm technique Fast-VESTAL successfully localized Broca's and Wernicke's areas in patients with tumors and epilepsy.[68]

Language Localization in Children

The verb-generation and picture-naming paradigms have been used successfully in children to localize expressive language function to the inferior frontal regions.[69,70] Receptive language lateralization using an auditory presentation task as described by Papanicolaou and colleagues[47] is well used in children and pediatric patients. This task has also been successfully used with children under sedation.[71] It appears that simple exposure to spectrally complex linguistic stimuli suffices to engage differentially the two hemispheres. Various other tasks have also been successfully used and are well described in a review by Pirmoradi and colleagues.[72]

Language-related evoked magnetic fields stimulation

Visually-presented words and objects are used to elicit language-related activity: In a verb-generation task, printed words are typically displayed for 2 seconds every 3 seconds. Stimuli consist of

100 concrete nouns (everyday words, selected for concreteness, and high frequency, ranging in length from four to eight letters). During each presentation the subject silently generates a verb that was linked to the noun (eg, book and read).[53] In a picture naming task, black-and-white line drawings of everyday objects (from Peabody's Picture Vocabulary Test) are visually displayed. During each presentation, the subject mentally identified the object and covertly named it.[53]

Continuous auditory word recognition tasks employ the presentation of a single word auditory stimulus with fixed or random inter-stimulus intervals, typically greater than 2 seconds. Stimuli are typically presented binaurally through inserted eartubes at normal listening levels (~60 dB above normal hearing levels), and patients are asked to either listen passively to the words or to covertly (silently) process the words or to indicate the presence of repeated word, depending on the particular protocol used. Examples of the word stimuli can be found in Papanicolaou and colleagues.[47]

Language-related evoked magnetic fields recording parameters
Recordings of responses to single-word stimuli are typically made with the bandpass set at 0.1 to 100 Hz and sampled at 508 Hz. Online averaging runs the risk of including trials with large movement artifacts and/or eye-blinks and should generally be avoided. Fifty to 100 trials are typically needed for averaging to provide a sufficiently clear signal.

Language-related evoked magnetic fields localization
Prior to analysis of the localization of the language responses, the data need to be inspected for movement and other artifacts. Then, averaging of 50 to 100 trials should provide a clear early response at approximately 100 milliseconds for either primary auditory or primary visual processing depending on the type of stimuli used. If a clear response is not seen in the average, the data should be inspected again for quality.

The data should be filtered 3 to 50 Hz. Inspection of the waveforms after the initial primary response at 100 milliseconds will display activity between 150 and 250 milliseconds, which is associated with receptive language and localizes to Wernicke area: superior temporal gyrus (Brodmann area 22), the angular gyrus (Brodmann 39), and the supramarginal gyrus (Brodmann 40). Expressive language response will be seen as peaks further down the waveform between 400 and 500 milliseconds and may extend to 750 milliseconds. These responses are associated with motor speech and localize to Broca area: pars opercularis and pars triangularis of the inferior frontal gyrus (Brodmann 44 and 45). The single equivalent current dipole (ECD) method has been widely used to determine the location of focal cortical sources involved in language processing.[63,73]

However, with advances being made in signal processing, many other MEG analytical techniques can also be used to identify language processing

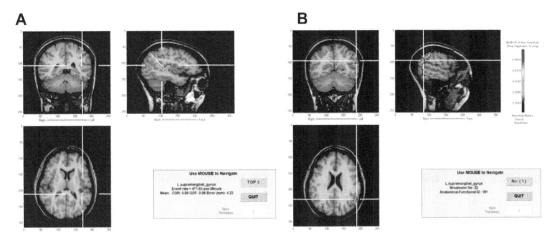

Fig. 6. A 55-year-old right-handed female with intractable localization related epilepsy had her LEF maps during a visual picture-naming task. (*A*) The ECD localization. (*B*) The current distribution technique (MR-FOCUSS). Note the ECD tends to localize deeper into the cortex than the current distribution technique. This is due to the MR-FOCUSS constraint to put the source in the gray matter (Subject ID IE2880).

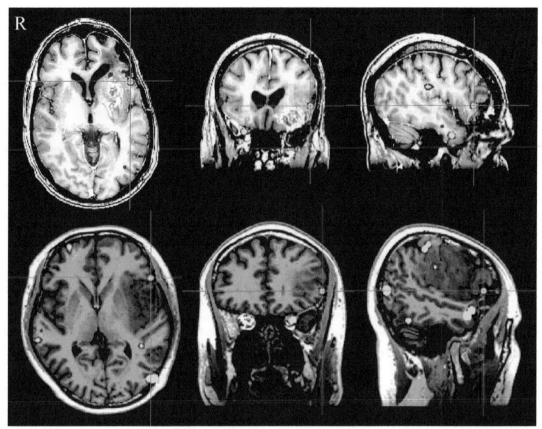

Fig. 7. Single subject–based MEG localization of Broca area (*green crosshairs*) in 2 subjects with large left frontal lobe tumors during object-naming task using Fast-VESTAL. In each subject, an *F* test was used to assess the statistical significance of the source magnitude (Root Mean Square [RMS] value) between 200 and 1000 milliseconds poststimulus interval and prestimulus baseline. (*From* Huang CW, Huang MX, Ji Z, et al. High-Resolution MEG Source Imaging Approach to accurately localize Broca's area in patients with Brain Tumor or Epilepsy. Clin Neurophysiol. 2016 May; 127(5):2308-16; with permission.)

areas in the brain, especially since language processing usually involves extended sources. Specifically, if the ECD fits do not perform as well as they did in this patient in Fig. 6, then using an advanced imaging technique may provide a better localization. Advanced MEG imaging alternatives such as current distribution techniques (MR- FOCUSS[67] or Fast-VESTAL[23]) and beamforming techniques have been used to localize the LEFs. These techniques can image extended areas of activity that are simultaneously active and that occur during language processing, whereas the single ECD can only image one small location at each millisecond in time. In Fig. 6 the second image shows the LEF result when MR-FOCUSS is applied to the same MEG data used for the ECD result from a picture-naming task.

A recent study by Huang and colleagues[68] used Fast-VESTAL[23] to identify Broca's area in patients with large left frontal tumors.[68] Fast-VESTAL localized Broca's area adjacent the tumors as seen for

example in Fig. 7. Besides accurately and reliably localizing Broca's and Wernicke's areas in patients with brain tumors and/or epilepsies, the Fast-VESTAL spatio-temporal L1 minimum norm analysis also showed that the Wernicke's area response significantly preceded the Broca's area response.

LEF maps are easily acquired at most MEG center locations. It is sometimes challenging for the analysis techniques to provide consistent results. The MEG centers with more experience using MEG imaging techniques beyond the single ECD (eg, MR-FOCUSS or Fast-VESTAL) have found that language mapping can be used to identify whether the LEF has undergone any functional reorganization because of a tumor or epileptogenic tissue.

SUMMARY

Noninvasive functional brain imaging with MEG is regularly used to map the eloquent cortex associated with somatosensory, motor, auditory, visual, and language processing prior to a surgical resection. Any cortical resection near an area of eloquent cortex should undergo an MEG study to determine if the functional areas have been reorganized due to the lesion/tumor or epileptogenic tissue. These localizations will also provide information on any possible deficits the patient may have after the resection. Most tasks are able to be performed in the pediatric population without too much trouble. To acquire an optimal MEG study for any of these modalities, the patient needs to be well rested and attending to the stimulation. Magnetoencephalography / Magnetic source imaging has the ability to localize eloquent cortices of interest noninvasively in patients, as well as identify displaced anatomic landmarks (central sulcus, sylvian fissure, etc.) and assist in optimizing the surgical trajectory for intraoperative navigation and surgical resection.

DISCLOSURE

The authors have nothing to disclose.

REFERENCES

1. Bardouille T, Power L, Lalancette M, et al. Variability and bias between magnetoencephalography systems in non-invasive localization of the primary somatosensory cortex. Clin Neurol Neurosurg 2018; 171:63–9.
2. Papanicolaou AC. Cllinical magnetoencephalography and magnetic source imaging. Cambridge (UK): Cambridge University Press; 2009.
3. Solomon J, Boe S, Bardouille T. Reliability for non-invasive somatosensory cortex localization: Implications for pre-surgical mapping. Clin Neurol Neurosurg 2015;139:224–9.
4. Willemse RB, Hillebrand A, Ronner HE, et al. Magnetoencephalographic study of hand and foot sensorimotor organization in 325 consecutive patients evaluated for tumor or epilepsy surgery. Neuroimage Clin 2015;10:46–53.
5. Ganslandt O, Buchfelder M, Hastreiter P, et al. Magnetic source imaging supports clinical decision making in glioma patients. Clin Neurol Neurosurg 2004;107(1):20–6.
6. Ishibashi H, Simos PG, Wheless JE, et al. Somatosensory evoked magnetic fields in hemimegalencephaly. Neurol Res 2002;24(5):459–62.
7. Schiffbauer H, Berger MS, Ferrari P, et al. Preoperative magnetic source imaging for brain tumor surgery: a quantitative comparison with intraoperative sensory and motor mapping. J Neurosurg 2002; 97(6):1333–42.
8. Korvenoja A, Kirveskari E, Aronen HJ, et al. Sensorimotor cortex localization: comparison of magnetoencephalography, functional MR imaging, and intraoperative cortical mapping. Radiology 2006; 241:213–22.
9. Ganslandt O, Fahlbusch R, Nimsky C, et al. Functional neuronavigation with magnetoencephalography: outcome in 50 patients with lesions around the motor cortex. J Neurosurg 1999; 91(1):73–9.
10. Castillo EM, Simos PG, Wheless JW, et al. Integrating sensory and motor mapping in a comprehensive MEG protocol: clinical validity and replicability. Neuroimage 2003;21:973–83.
11. Lin YY, Shih YH, Chang KP, et al. MEG localization of rolandic spikes with respect to SI and SII cortices in benign rolandic epilepsy. Neuroimage 2003;20(4):2051–6.
12. Romstöck J, Fahlbusch R, Ganslandt O, et al. Localisation of the sensorimotor cortex during surgery for brain tumours: feasibility and waveform patterns of somatosensory evoked potentials. J Neurol Neurosurg Psychiatry 2002;72(2):221–9.
13. Pihko E, Nevalainen P, Stephen J, et al. Maturation of somatosensory cortical processing from birth to adulthood revealed by magnetoencephalography. Clin Neurophysiol 2009;120(8):1552–61.
14. Chuang NA, Otsubo H, Pang EW, et al. Pediatric magnetoencephalography and magnetic source imaging. Neuroimaging Clin N Am 2006;16(1): 193–210. ix-x.
15. Sharma R, Pang EW, Mohamed I, et al. Magnetoencephalography in children: routine clinical protocol for intractable epilepsy at the Hospital for Sick Children. International Congress Series 2007;1300: 685–8.
16. Bercovici E, Pang EW, Sharma R, et al. Somatosensory-evoked fields on magnetoencephalography for epilepsy infants younger than 4 years with total intravenous anesthesia. Clin Neurophysiol 2008;119(6): 1328–34.
17. Kassubek J, Stippich C, Sörös P, et al. A motor field source localization protocol using magnetoencephalography. Biomedical Engineering/Biomedizinische Technik 2009;41(1):334–5.
18. Cheyne D, Bakhtazad L, Gaetz W. Spatiotemporal mapping of cortical activity accompanying voluntary movements using an event-related beamforming approach. Hum Brain Mapp 2006;27:213–29.
19. Nagamine T, Kajola M, Salmelin R, et al. Movement-related slow cortical magnetic fields and changes of spontaneous MEG- and EEG-brain rhythms. Electroencephalogr Clin Neurophysiol 1996;99(3): 274–86.
20. Cheyne D, Kristeva R, Deecke L. Homuncular organization of human motor cortex as indicated by neuromagnetic recordings. Neurosci Lett 1991;122(1): 17–20.

21. Kristeva-Feige R, Rossi S, Pizzella V, et al. Changes in movement-related brain activity during transient deafferentation: a neuromagnetic study. Brain Res 1996;714(1-2):201–8.

22. Hoshiyama M, Kakigi R, Berg P, et al. Identification of motor and sensory brain activities during unilateral finger movement: spatiotemporal source analysis of movement-associated magnetic fields. Exp Brain Res 1997;115(1):6–14.

23. Huang M-X, Huang CW, Robb A, et al. MEG source imaging method using fast L1 minimum-norm and its applications to signals with brain noise and human resting-state source amplitude images. NeuroImage 2014;84:585–604.

24. Zimmermann M, Rössler K, Kaltenhäuser M, et al. Comparative fMRI and MEG localization of cortical sensorimotor function: bimodal mapping supports motor area reorganization in glioma patients. PLoS One 2019;14:e0213371.

25. Cheyne D, Jobst C, Tesan G, et al. Movement-related neuromagnetic fields in preschool age children. Hum Brain Mapp 2014;35(9):4858–75.

26. Gaetz W, Cheyne D, Rutka JT, et al. Presurgical localization of primary motor cortex in pediatric patients with brain lesions by the use of spatially filtered magnetoencephalography. Neurosurgery 2009;64:177–85.

27. Jacobson G. Magnetoencephalographic studies of auditory system function. J Clin Neurophysiol 1994;11(3):343–64.

28. Parkkonen L, Fujiki N, Mäkelä J. Sources of auditory brainstem responses revisited: contribution by magnetoencephalography. Hum Brain Mapp 2009;30:1772–82.

29. Nakasato N, Fujita S, Seki K, et al. Functional localization of bilateral auditory cortices using an MRI-linked whole head magnetoencephalography (MEG) system. Electroencephalogr Clin Neurophysiol 1995;94(3):183–90.

30. Verkindt C, Bertrand O, Perrin F, et al. Tonotopic organization of the human auditory cortex: N100 topography and multiple dipole model analysis. Electroencephalogr Clin Neurophysiol 1995;96(2):143–56.

31. Pantev C, Bertrand O, Eulitz C, et al. Specific somatotopic organizations of different areas of the human auditory cortex revealed by simultaneous magnetic and electric recordings. Electroencephalogr Clin Neurophysiol 1995;94:26–40.

32. Nakasato N, Kumabe T, Kanno A, et al. Neuromagnetic evaluation of cortical auditory function in patients with temporal lobe tumors. J Neurosurg 1997;86:610–8.

33. Kanno A, Nakasato N, Murayama N, et al. Middle and long latency peak sources in auditory evoked magnetic fields for tone bursts in humans. Neurosci Lett 2000;293(3):187–90.

34. Paetau R, Ahonen A, Salonen O, et al. Auditory evoked magnetic fields to tones and pseudowords in healthy children and adults. J Clin Neurophysiol 1995;12(2):177–85.

35. Takeshita K, Nagamine T, Thuy DH, et al. Maturational change of parallel auditory processing in school-aged children revealed by simultaneous recording of magnetic and electric cortical responses. Clin Neurophysiol 2002;113(9):1470–84.

36. Holst M, Eswaran H, Lowery C, et al. Development of auditory evoked fields in human fetuses and newborns: a longitudinal MEG study. Clin Neurophysiol 2005;116(8):1949–55.

37. Chen WT, Ko YC, Liao KK, et al. Optimal check size and reversal rate to elicit pattern-reversal MEG responses. Can J Neurol Sci 2005;32:218–24.

38. Harding GF, Armstrong RA, Janday B. Visual evoked electrical and magnetic response to half-field stimulation using pattern reversal stimulation. Ophthalmic Physiol Opt 1992;12:171–4.

39. Alberstone CD, Skirboll SL, Benzel EC, et al. Magnetic source imaging and brain surgery: presurgical and intraoperative planning in 26 patients. J Neurosurg 2000;92(1):79–90.

40. Inoue T, Fujimura M, Kumabe T, et al. Combined three-dimensional anisotropy contrast imaging and magnetoencephalography guidance to preserve visual function in a patient with an occipital lobe tumor. Minim Invasive Neurosurg 2004;47(4):249–52.

41. Barnikol UB, Amunts K, Dammers J, et al. Pattern reversal visual evoked responses of V1/V2 and V5/MT as revealed by MEG combined with probabilistic cytoarchitectonic maps. Neuroimage 2006;31(1):86–108.

42. Hashimoto T, Kashii S, Kikuchi M, et al. Temporal profile of visual evoked responses to pattern-reversal stimulation analyzed with a whole-head magnetometer. Exp Brain Res 1999;125(3):375–82.

43. Nakamura M, Kakigi R, Okusa T, et al. Effects of check size on pattern reversal visual evoked magnetic field and potential. Brain Res 2000;872(1-2):77–86.

44. Grover KM, Bowyer SM, Rock J, et al. Retrospective review of MEG visual evoked hemifield responses prior to resection of temporo-parieto-occipital lesions. Neurooncol 2006;22(2):161–6.

45. Chen Y, Xiang J, Kirtman EG, et al. Neuromagnetic biomarkers of visuocortical development in healthy children. Clin Neurophysiol 2010;121(9):1555–62.

46. Castillo EM, Simos PG, Venkataraman V, et al. Mapping of expressive language cortex using magnetic source imaging. Neurocase 2001;7:419–22.

47. Papanicolaou AC, Simos PG, Castillo EM, et al. Magnetocephalography: a noninvasive alternative to the Wada procedure. J Neurosurg 2004;100:867–76.

48. Bowyer SM, Moran JE, Weiland BJ, et al. Language Laterality Determined by MEG Mapping with MR-FOCUSS. Epilepsy & Behavior 2005;6:235–41.

49. Papanicolaou AC, Simos PG, Breier JI, et al. Magnetoencephalographic mapping of the language-specific cortex. Journal of Neurosurgery 1999;90(1): 85–93.

50. Breier JI, Simos PG, Zouridakis G, et al. Lateralization of activity associated with language function using magnetoencephalography: a reliability study. J Clin Neurophysiol 2000;17(5):503–10.

51. Breier JI, Simos PG, Wheless JW, et al. Language dominance in children as determined by magnetic source imaging and the intracarotid amobarbital procedure: a comparison. J Child Neurol 2001;16: 124–30.

52. Maestú F, Ortiz T, Fernandez A, et al. Spanish language mapping using MEG: a validation study. Neuroimage 2002;17(3):1579–86.

53. Bowyer SM, Moran JE, Mason KM, et al. MEG localization of language-specific cortex utilizing MR-FOCUSS. Neurology 2004;62(12):2247–55.

54. Hirata M, Kato A, Taniguchi M, et al. Determination of language dominance with synthetic aperture magnetometry: comparison with the Wada test. Neuroimage 2004;23(1):46–53.

55. Kamada K, Sawamura Y, Takeuchi F, et al. Expressive and receptive language areas determined by non-invasive reliable methods using functional magnetic resonance imaging and magnetoencephalography. Neurosurgery 2007;60:296–306.

56. McDonald CR, Thesen T, Hagler DJ Jr, et al. Distributed source modeling of language with magnetoencephalography: application to patients with intractable epilepsy. Epilepsia 2009;50(10): 2256–66.

57. Hirata M, Goto T, Barnes G, et al. Language dominance and mapping based on neuromagnetic oscillatory changes: comparison with invasive procedures. J Neurosurg 2010;112(3):528–38.

58. Findlay AM, Ambrose JB, Cahn-Weiner DA, et al. Dynamics of hemispheric dominance for language assessed by magnetoencephalographic imaging. Ann Neurol 2012;71(5):668–86.

59. Tanaka N, Liu H, Reinsberger C, et al. Language lateralization represented by spatiotemporal mapping of magnetoencephalography. AJNR Am J Neuroradiol 2013;34(3):558–63.

60. Doss RC, Zhang W, Risse GL, et al. Lateralizing language with magnetic source imaging: validation based on the Wada test. Epilepsia 2009;50(10): 2242–8.

61. Warren JE, Crinion JT, Lambon Ralph MA, et al. Anterior temporal lobe connectivity correlates with functional outcome after aphasic stroke. Brain 2009;132:3428–42.

62. Hillis AE, Wityk RJ, Tuffiash E, et al. Hypoperfusion of Wernicke's area predicts severity of semantic deficit in acute stroke. Ann Neurol 2001;50(5):561–6.

63. Simos PG, Castillo EM, Fletcher JM, et al. Mapping of receptive language cortex in bilingual volunteers by using magnetic source imaging. J Neurosurg 2001;95(1):76–81.

64. Castillo EM, Breier JI, Wheless JW, et al. Contributions of direct cortical stimulation and MEG recordings to identify "essential" language cortex. Epilepsia 2005;46(324).

65. Hillis AE, Kleinman JT, Newhart M, et al. Restoring cerebral blood flow reveals neural regions critical for naming. J Neurosci 2006;26(31):8069–73.

66. Kober H, Möller M, Nimsky C, et al. New approach to localize speech relevant brain areas and hemispheric dominance using spatially filtered magnetoencephalography. Hum Brain Mapp 2001;14(4): 236–50.

67. Moran JE, Bowyer S, Tepley N. Multi-Resolution FOCUSS: A source imaging technique applied to MEG data. Brain Topography 2005;18(1):1–17.

68. Huang CW, Huang M-X, Ji Z, et al. High-resolution MEG source imaging approach to accurately localize Broca's area in patients with brain tumor or epilepsy. Clin Neurophysiol 2016;127: 2308–16.

69. Foley E, Cross JH, Thai NJ, et al. MEG assessment of expressive language in children evaluated for epilepsy surgery. Brain Topogr 2019;32(3): 492–503.

70. Pang EW, Wang F, Malone M, et al. Localization of Broca's area using verb generation tasks in the MEG: validation against fMRI. Neurosci Lett 2011; 490(3):215–9.

71. Rezaie R, Narayana S, Schiller K, et al. Assessment of hemispheric dominance for receptive language in pediatric patients under sedation using magnetoencephalography. Front Hum Neurosci 2014;8:657.

72. Pirmoradi M, Béland R, Nguyen DK, et al. Language tasks used for the presurgical assessment of epileptic patients with MEG. Epileptic Disord 2010; 1292:97–108.

73. Simos PG, Breier JI, Zouridakis G, et al. Identification of language-specific brain activity using magnetoencephalography. J Clin Exp Neuropsychol 1998; 20(5):706–22.

Magnetoencephalography for Mild Traumatic Brain Injury and Posttraumatic Stress Disorder

Mingxiong Huang, PhD[a], Jeffrey David Lewine, PhD[b], Roland R. Lee, MD[a],*

KEYWORDS

- Traumatic brain injury • Slow wave • Gamma wave • GABA-ergic • Posttraumatic stress disorder
- Functional connectivity

KEY POINTS

- MEG can provide sensitive biomarkers for detecting abnormalities in mTBI and PTSD.
- MEG frequently reveals abnormal slow-wave activity related to cortical deafferentation in mTBI.
- Following mTBI, MEG may also demonstrate hyperactivity in the gamma-band which is believed to reflect disruption of normal GABA-ergic inhibitory mechanisms
- TBI-related disruption of axonal pathways may also be identified through MEG-based measures of functional connectivity.
- TBI-related disruption of gray and white matter may manifest as abnormalities in MEG event-related fields.

OVERVIEW OF HEAD TRAUMA AND TRAUMATIC BRAIN INJURY

Each year more than 2.5 million people sustain a head trauma in the United States alone.[1,2] More than 500,000 of these persons require hospitalization, with 90,000 of the survivors afflicted with the long-term sequelae of these injuries.[3,4] The estimated cost for the care of these head trauma victims approaches $50 billion per year. Posttraumatic symptoms of moderate and severe trauma may include neurologic impairment and/or persistent symptoms in somatic, psychiatric-behavioral, and cognitive domains.[5–10] Somatic symptoms, including headache, fatigue, sensory changes, balance problems, and sleep disturbance, are common following head trauma, as are symptoms of psychiatric-behavioral disturbance related to increased depression, anxiety, posttraumatic stress disorder (PTSD), irritability,

and inappropriate behaviors. Cognitive impairments may also be reported following head trauma, especially with respect to problems in memory, attention, executive functioning, processing speed, and multitasking. Immediately after mild head trauma, many victims also complain of similar symptoms, but in most cases these symptoms subside within a few weeks. However, even when there is no loss of consciousness, 10% to 30% of individuals who suffer minor head trauma still report postconcussive problems several years after the incident.[6,7,11–18]

Given that mild head trauma accounts for more than 70% of all cases of head trauma, in the United States, there are more than 200,000 new civilian patients each year with persistent postconcussive symptoms (PCS) after mild trauma.[1,19] Mild head trauma is also especially problematic in present day military settings, where blast waves can

[a] Department of Radiology, University of California, San Diego and VA San Diego, UCSD Radiology Imaging Lab, 3510 Dunhill Street, San Diego, CA 92121, USA; [b] The Mind Research Network, 1101 Yale Boulevard, Albuquerque, NM 87106, USA
* Corresponding author.
E-mail address: RRLEE@UCSD.EDU

Neuroimag Clin N Am 30 (2020) 175–192
https://doi.org/10.1016/j.nic.2020.02.003
1052-5149/20/Published by Elsevier Inc.

induce head trauma over an extended area. Current data indicate that almost 400,000 American service members have suffered mild head trauma during recent conflicts in the Middle East. Mild head trauma is therefore a significant clinical problem in its own right, and an understanding of the neurobiological consequences of head trauma is becoming of increasing interest in general medicine, especially because the deleterious effects of head trauma and concussions appear to be cumulative,[20,21] and even a single episode of mild head trauma may convey increased risk for certain other medical conditions (eg, Alzheimer dementia[22–27]).

Available human and animal neuroscientific data indicate that traumatic brain injury (TBI) is a potential consequence of the initial primary mechanical forces of head trauma, and the result of subsequent damage caused by a secondary injury cascade, which comes into play during the minutes, hours, days, weeks, and even months following an initial traumatic event. TBI is a process, not an event.[28] Dependent on the magnitude of the initial mechanical forces, primary damage may include subdural and subarachnoid hematoma, contusions to cortical regions, intraparenchymal hemorrhage, and/or axonal shearing and diffuse axonal injury (DAI). The secondary injury cascade is characterized by changes in brain chemistry (neurotransmitter release and excitotoxicity), hemodynamic changes, changes in glucose metabolism, breakdown of the blood-brain barrier, and a neuroinflammatory response.[29] The secondary cascade can be triggered by even mild low-impact events, and it may also lead to cell death and axonal damage. Indeed, in some cases, secondary damage is more significant and extensive than the primary damage. It is presently unknown why some individuals recover fully from substantial blows to the head, whereas others may dramatically decompensate from relatively low-level mechanical forces,[30] but there is growing suspicion that the situation is mostly a reflection of how secondary (rather than primary) injury processes ultimately impact each individual's brain.

THE NEED FOR ADVANCED IMAGING AND ELECTROPHYSIOLOGICAL METHODS

Optimized treatment strategies for mild traumatic brain injury (mTBI) have been difficult to develop in part because there is usually only very limited information on the loci and mechanisms of injury. Therefore, many have turned toward advanced neuroscience methods for understanding TBI in animal and human models. Although the animal data are clear that even very low-level traumatic forces can lead to negative neurobiological and behavioral consequences, the human situation with respect to mTBI remains somewhat controversial, especially because routine structural imaging (computed tomography and MR imaging) generally fails to reveal any persistent abnormalities in the victims of mild head trauma.[9,31,32] As a result of this observation, some postulate that persistent complaints following mild head trauma are almost always a reflection of premorbid psychopathology or even fabrications motivated by a desire to avoid work or to seek financial gain through legal actions.[33–35] However, recently available advanced imaging procedures repeatedly demonstrate that persistent symptoms sometimes truly reflect an actual injury to the brain (ie, TBI). Advanced methods of increasing interest include MR imaging–based volumetric and diffusion-weighted imaging,[36–39] metabolic methods such as positron emission tomography (PET) and single-photon emission computed tomography (SPECT),[40–43] and electrophysiological techniques, including electroencephalogram (EEG) and magnetoencephalography (MEG).[44–53]

In considering the utility of each of these methods, attention must be given to sensitivity, specificity, and positive and negative predictive value. For example, much recent work has focused on the use of diffusion tensor imaging (DTI) for the identification of axonal damage related to head trauma. Several lines of data converge to indicate that axonal fibers are particularly vulnerable to traumatic forces (eg, Ref.[54]) with trauma resulting in diffuse axonal damage and network disruption.[55,56] On the one hand, available data do indeed indicate that DTI is substantially more sensitive to TBI than traditional routine clinical MR imaging, which generally reveals abnormalities in less than 10% of mTBI cases, even in the acute period. In the chronic period, the sensitivity of routine MR imaging drops to <5%.[50,57] On the other hand, the sensitivity of DTI to mTBI at the individual subject level is generally reported to be relatively low (20%–30%) in both acute and chronic periods.[58–60]

DTI also has potential issues with respect to specificity, because many other neurologic and psychiatric conditions are also associated with abnormal DTI metrics (eg, Refs.[61,62]). It is not sufficient to simply demonstrate that a method distinguishes TBI clients from control subjects with no history of neurologic or psychiatric disease. Specificity with respect to a wide range of common clinical conditions (eg, depression, substance use disorder, migraines) is needed. DTI analyses are not presently of utility as stand-alone tests of the presence of TBI. The information must always be considered with the context of a subject's medical history, timeline, and symptom development, and other neurologic, psychiatric, psychological, radiologic, and electrophysiologic evaluations. At present, most professional organizations do not advocate for the use of DTI in the *routine clinical* evaluation of mTBI in individual patients, and this is presently appropriate (eg, Radiological Society of North America Statement on TBI Imaging, September 13, 2018, https://www.rsna.org/uploadedFiles/RSNA/Content/Role_based_pages/Media/RSNA-TBI-Position-Statement.pdf). However, this does not mean that the method is not scientifically valid, or that it might not be of high utility in a particular case (especially within a forensic setting). Rather, it is merely an indication that performing DTI routinely in the acute setting of an mTBI is usually of little value for guiding patient management.

Given that both primary and secondary injury mechanisms in head trauma often affect the mechanisms that support the generation, transmission, and processing of electrophysiological signals within and between brain regions, there is good reason to believe (and mounting data to support) the view that MEG, with its high spatial and temporal resolution and direct sensitivity to electrophysiological activity, is one of the best techniques for observing trauma-induced disruption of the brain. This article focuses on resting-state activity profiles in MEG as potential biomarkers of TBI-induced dysfunction.

MAGNETOENCEPHALOGRAPHY RESTING STATE DATA: SLOW WAVES

With respect to resting state data, TBI-related axonal disruption is likely to perturb both the profile of intrinsic background rhythms and measures of functional connectivity (FC) between brain regions (especially with respect to interhemispheric relationships, given the known sensitivity of the corpus callosum to traumatic forces). In considering this, it is important to note that TBI-related axonal disruption is not restricted to long fiber tracts. Rather, damage may be seen both in projection pathways and with respect to local interconnections within the gray matter (GM),[63] with additional damage to GM neurons and glia also possible,[64] with some evidence of selective vulnerability of GABA-ergic interneurons. From a neurophysiological perspective, several TBI-related changes to intrinsic rhythms are expected, including an increase in abnormal low-frequency magnetic activity in the delta range, and an increase in abnormal high-frequency magnetic activity in the gamma- and high beta-bands.

Prior animal studies have established a clear connection between brain lesions and pathologic slow-wave (1–4 Hz) generation in cortex. For example, several studies demonstrate that placement of lesions disrupting thalamocortical projections in the subcortical white matter (WM) give rise to the generation of focal slow waves in the overlying cortex.[65,66] Disruption of ascending cholinergic fibers can also induce slow waves in deafferented cortical regions.[67,68] In both the EEG and the MEG, abnormal delta activity may also be seen when tissue becomes ischemic, either by disruption of blood flow as in a stroke or through compression as is seen with space-occupying tumors (EEG[69,70]; MEG[71,72]). Focal slowing may also be seen in cases of epilepsy, and whenever there are regions of frank encephalomalacia.[73]

With respect to head trauma, both axonal damage and direct GM damage can give rise to focal slow waves. It should be noted that slow waves can be seen under certain normal circumstances (eg, during certain phases of drowsiness and sleep), and they can be induced by certain medications, but the slow waves in these circumstances are generally not focal. In the MEG, focal, pathologic slow waves are well modeled by simple dipoles, whereas nonpathologic slow waves of sleep and drowsiness are multifocal or arise from large extended brain regions that are not adequately modeled by single dipoles.[74]

Fig. 1 illustrates a general lack of MEG slow waves in an awake healthy control subject versus a prominence of delta activity in a patient with an intracranial lesion (in this case, a stroke). In the stroke patient, most of the slow waves have complicated magnetic field patterns that are poorly modeled by a dipole source. However, some slow waves are highly dipolar. Fig. 2 shows that consideration of all slow waves provides only limited information on the location of pathologic condition, whereas dipolar slow waves selectively cluster along the margins of demonstrable lesions. Fig. 3 shows an explicit example from a head trauma patient with a clear region of TBI in the left frontal lobe. Dipolar slow-wave analyses demonstrate the presence of dysfunction along the margins of the lesion.

The early observations that dipolar slow waves were selectively generated at regions of clear structural pathologic condition provided the foundation for subsequent studies in mTBI, where structural MR imaging rarely reveals gross pathologic condition. The rationale was that dipolar slow waves might be able to indicate focal pathophysiology even in cases where the relevant structural damage was too subtle to be seen on routine

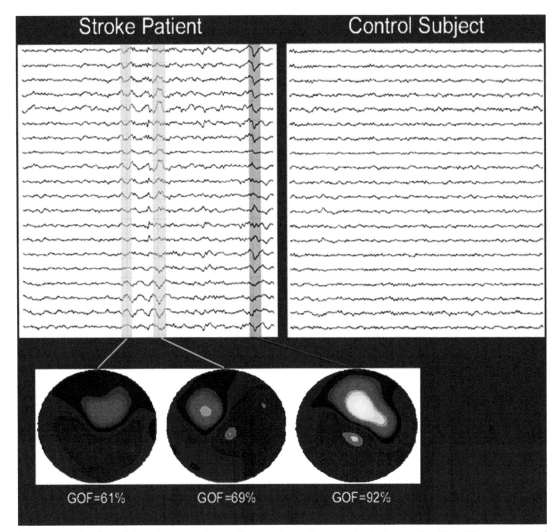

Fig. 1. Example of MEG data from a patient with a stroke and a neurotypical control subject. The upper panels show 5 seconds of data from representative channels. For neurotypical control subjects, slow waves are generally not seen at all, except during drowsiness or sleep. In contrast, patients with intracranial pathologic condition often show substantial activity in the delta range. Most slow waves, even in patients with pathologic condition, are multifocal, and poorly modeled by single dipoles, as illustrated in the lower isofield contour maps (with displayed goodness-of-fit [GOF] for a single dipole model). However, some slow waves (eg, the transient in *red*) have quite focal generation (as indicated by a dipolar field pattern and high GOF).

clinical MR imaging. This notion was subsequently borne out by the seminal studies of Lewine and colleagues,[50,51] demonstrating a high rate of dipolar slow-wave activity in mTBI patients without clear lesions.

As described in Lewine and colleagues,[50] procedures for dipolar slow-wave analyses using Neuromag-306 channel systems are all objective. Briefly, following artifact removal, data are filtered between 1 and 6 Hz, and large-amplitude slow waves (>200 fT on at least 1 magnetometer channel) are identified. A 50-millisecond window about the peak of each slow wave is evaluated with a single equivalent current dipole fit every 10 milliseconds. The single best fit within each event window is then retained for further consideration. If the goodness of fit for the dipole model is greater than 0.8 with only planar sensors included during the fitting procedure (or >0.65 with all 306 channels included), the dipole is considered a viable model, and its spatial parameters are noted. A spatial clustering algorithm is then used to determine for each viable dipole how many neighbor dipoles are seen within a $2 \times 2 \times 2$-cm^3 region. If this value exceeds 1 dipole per minute of recording time, then all members of the dipole cluster are

All Slow Waves

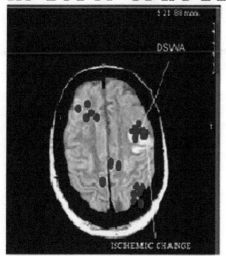

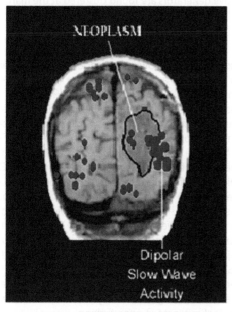

Only Highly Dipolar Slow Waves

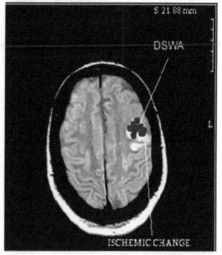

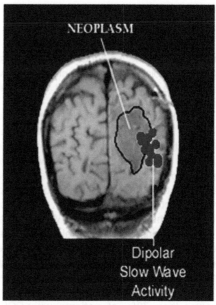

Fig. 2. Although the general presence of delta activity is often a sign of some type of pathologic condition (except during drowsiness or sleep, or in the presence of certain psychoactive compounds), source modeling of all slow waves reveals a poor relationship between the spatial distribution of sources (*red circles*) and regions of clear pathologic condition (*left panels*). In contrast, if only highly dipolar slow-wave activity (DSWA) is considered, the sources cluster at regions of pathologic condition and are not seen elsewhere in the brain (*right panels*).

retained and plotted on spatially aligned MR imaging to generate magnetic source localization images. That is, in order for a region to be considered a generator of pathologic slow waves, it must be responsible for generation of multiple events. Single, isolated slow waves are not clear indicators of pathophysiology. These values have been identified as optimal for distinguishing patients with mTBI patients with persistent PCS and neurotypical controls. **Table 1** provides

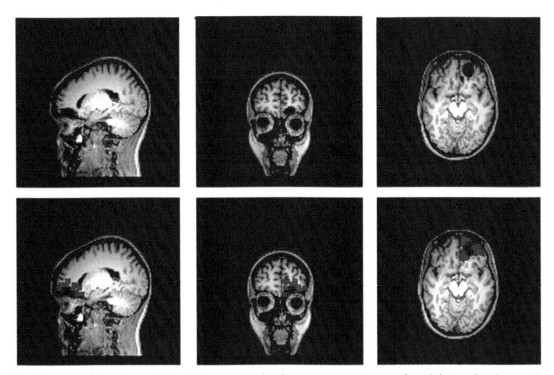

Fig. 3. In cases of clear traumatic brain damage, dipolar slow-wave generators are found clustered at the margins of lesioned tissues as shown in the lower magnetic source localization images, where each red box indicates the location of the generator of a single dipolar slow-wave transient.

information on the incidence of the presence of 1 or more dipolar slow source clusters for various populations of particular interest when evaluating TBI.

The data reveal several important observations. First, the "false positive" incidence of dipolar slow-wave activity in neurotypical control subjects is quite low (~6%), and when slow waves are seen in control subjects, they are almost always restricted to the occipital region (only 1% of control subjects show slow-wave source clusters outside of the occipital lobes). Within the studied TBI populations, there is a relationship between severity of symptoms/injury severity and the presence of slow waves. Subjects with a history of mTBI, but without current persistent PCS generally do not show dipolar slow-wave activity, whereas greater than 70% of patients with PCS show slow-wave source clusters. It is also noteworthy that the sensitivity of MEG to pathophysiology in mTBI is much higher than that seen for conventional structural MR imaging, clinical EEG, and clinical SPECT (MEG, 71.5%; MR imaging, 13.3%; EEG, 20.6%; SPECT, 4%; see Ref.[50]).

With respect to specific PCS, expected relationships are seen between dipole cluster locations and particular symptoms. That is, subjects with temporal slowing are associated with memory deficits; parietal slowing is associated with attention problems, and frontal slowing is associated with problems in executive function.[50]

As an alternative to dipole-based analyses, Huang and colleagues,[47,48] as described in subsequent sections, have been exploring the utility of the VESTAL distributed source model for identification of pathophysiology in patients with mTBI. Available data suggest that this approach may be even more sensitive to the presence of pathophysiology in mTBI than the dipole approach, and it may have higher specificity, at least with respect to false positive identifications in control subjects. At present, differential specificity of the VESTAL approach with respect to many of the conditions presented in **Table 1** needs to be determined, but the high specificity with respect to neurotypical subjects is encouraging.

Using VESTAL, Huang and colleagues[47,48] have demonstrated that MEG delta-wave source imaging detects abnormal delta-waves with ~85% sensitivity in patients with persistent PCS in chronic and subacute phases of mTBI.[75] **Fig. 4** shows the MEG slow-wave measures (Z_{cmax} values [see Ref.[47]]) obtained from MEG source magnitude source imaging, plotted separately for (a) 79 healthy control subjects, (b) 36 individuals with mild blast-induced TBI, and (c) 48 individuals

Table 1
Data on the incidence of clusters of dipolar slow-wave sources in various populations

Type of Subject	Number of Subjects	% with Dipolar Slow Waves
Neurotypical control	214	6.1[a]
History of mTBI but no current PCS	33	15.2
History of mTBI with PCS	242	71.5
History of moderate TBI with PCS	42	83.3
PTSD with no TBI	46	13.0
Alcohol use disorder	14	28.5[b]
Active major depressive disorder	25	16.0
Active anxiety disorder	18	16.7
Attention-deficit/ hyperactivity disorder	14	14.3

Note that all subjects reported in this table are older than 8 y of age. Preliminary data indicate that the baseline rate of slow-wave activity approaches 15% to 20% in younger control children (ages 3–7). It is also noteworthy that the incidence of dipolar slow-wave activity does not substantially increase with normal aging up through 80 y of age, although older patients with clear signs of mild cognitive impairment or clear Alzheimer disease do show an increased incidence of slowing (~17% and 23%, respectively).

[a] When slow waves are present for control subjects, there is typically only a single cluster in the occipital region.

[b] All subjects with alcohol use disorders that showed slow-wave source clusters had clear evidence of global cortical atrophy.

with mild nonblast TBI. The optimal cutoff (threshold) for Z_{cmax} was obtained from the Youden's index curve (embedded plot in **Fig. 4**) using 79 healthy controls and 84 mTBI patients (blast plus nonblast). A more conservative cutoff value of 2.50 was chosen here (solid lines), which corresponded to specificity of 100% (ie, 0 false positive rate, no healthy control subjects showed Z_{cmax} value above this threshold). With this threshold (solid horizontal line in **Fig. 4**), the positive detection rates (ie, sensitivity values) were 86.1%, 83.3%, and 84.5% for blast-induced, nonblast, and combined (blast-induced plus nonblast) mTBI groups, respectively.

There was minimal overlap of the Z_{cmax} values between each TBI group and the healthy control group, with the patients in all TBI groups showing markedly higher slow-wave Z_{cmax} values than the healthy control subjects. Such results provide the

foundation for assessing abnormality in mTBI using MEG slow-wave source imaging on a single-subject basis. **Fig. 5** shows the abnormal MEG slow-wave source images in 8 representative mTBI subjects obtained using Fast-VESTAL algorithm (see Matti Hämäläinen and colleagues' article, "MEG Signal Processing, Forward Modeling, MEG Inverse Source Imaging, and Coherence Analysis," in this issue and Ref.[76]). As is found for dipole analyses, the location of generators of MEG slow-wave sources is heterogeneous across subjects, which is largely due to the nature of head trauma, with variable sites of impact and mechanical dynamics across patients.

Although the location of slow-wave generation is highly heterogeneous in locations across mTBI patients, analysis has been performed to identify common brain areas that likely generate VESTAL-identified abnormal MEG slow-wave activity in mTBI. The percent likelihood of abnormal MEG slow-wave generation revealed that the overall percent likelihood level from any specific brain area was low (5%–15%). However, the following areas showed higher likelihood than the rest of the brain for generating abnormal slow-waves: bilateral dorsolateral prefrontal cortex (DLPFC), bilateral ventral lateral prefrontal cortex, bilateral frontal pole (FP), right orbitofrontal cortex (OFC), left inferior-lateral-posterior parietal lobe, bilateral inferior temporal lobes, right hippocampus, and bilateral cerebella.[47]

MAGNETOENCEPHALOGRAPHY RESTING STATE DATA: GAMMA-BAND ACTIVITY

Animal and human data converge to indicate that primary traumatic forces and secondary injury cascades triggered by head trauma can cause GM damage, with some studies suggesting special vulnerability of GABA-ergic inhibitory interneurons. Trauma may cause damage specifically near the soma of the parvalbumin-positive (PV$^+$) interneurons (see references in Ref.[63]), and it may degrade the perineuronal net, which is a specialized extracellular structure enwrapping cortical PV$^+$ inhibitory interneurons.[77] Fast-spiking PV$^+$ inhibitory interneurons are the most common type of GABA-ergic cells that express the calcium-binding protein PV$^+$ and receive N-methyl-D-aspartate–dependent excitatory input from pyramidal cells.[78,79] Fast-spiking PV$^+$ interneurons regulate the activity of neural networks through GABA-ergic inhibition of local excitatory neurons and generate gamma oscillations (30–80 Hz) through synchronous activity.[78,80–83] Animal studies demonstrate that dysfunction or injury to PV$^+$ interneurons causes disinhibition in the neural

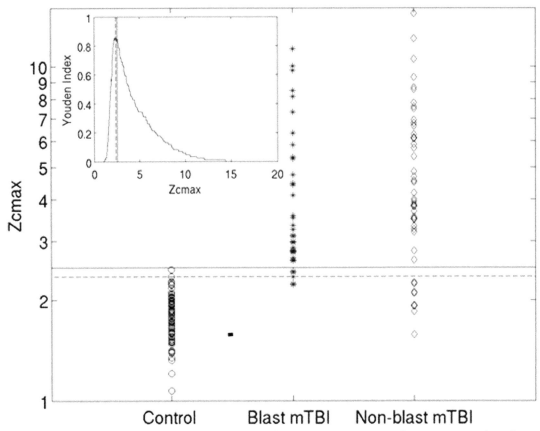

Fig. 4. MEG slow-wave measures (Z_{cmax} values) obtained from MEG source imaging for 1 to 4 Hz are plotted separately for (1) healthy control, (2) mild blast-induced TBI, and (3) mild non-blast-induced TBI, groups respectively. The embedded plot: the Youden index, is plotted as a function of the Z_{cmax} cutoff. (*From* Huang, M.-X., Nichols, S., Baker, D.G., et al. Single-subject-based whole-brain MEG slow-wave imaging approach for detecting abnormality in patients with mild traumatic brain injury. NeuroImage Clin. 2014; 5, p. 109–119; with permission. (Figure 2 in original) https://doi.org/10.1016/j.nicl.2014.06.004.)

network by (1) directly eliminating synchronized gamma-band (30–80 Hz) signals that are normally evoked by stimuli during the poststimulus interval,[78,84,85] and (2) upregulating spontaneous gamma (and maybe beta) activity, because of absent inhibition of excitatory neurons.[78,84–87]

Synchronized gamma oscillatory activity occurs throughout the cortex, in support of information processing during cognition.[88] In humans with TBI, synchronized gamma signals are abnormal during evoked EEG or MEG recordings. It was found that during working memory, evoked gamma-band MEG responses in individuals with mTBI were reduced in posterior DLPFC, a component of the working memory network, but increased in the FP and anterior DLPFC.[89] During working memory retention, gamma-band FC of posterior regions was aberrantly increased in individuals with TBI or major depressive disorder following TBI.[90] Abnormally delayed gamma-

band (40 Hz) EEG latency in TBI patients was also observed during an auditory oddball task.[91] Interestingly, reduced synchronization of gamma-band signals is found in evoked-MEG responses to somatosensory stimuli in human immunodeficiency virus patients,[92] and in evoked-EEG responses to auditory stimuli in schizophrenia.[93,94] Importantly, both disorders exhibit injury to GABA-ergic interneurons.[78,95]

A recent study by Huang and colleagues[46] investigated spontaneous gamma-band MEG source imaging during resting-state MEG recordings in individuals with persistent postconcussive symptoms in the chronic period following blast-related mTBI.[46] Participants included 25 symptomatic individuals with chronic combat-related blast mTBI, and 35 healthy controls with similar combat experiences. MEG source images were obtained using the Fast-VESTAL algorithm (see Matti Hämäläinen and colleagues' article, "MEG

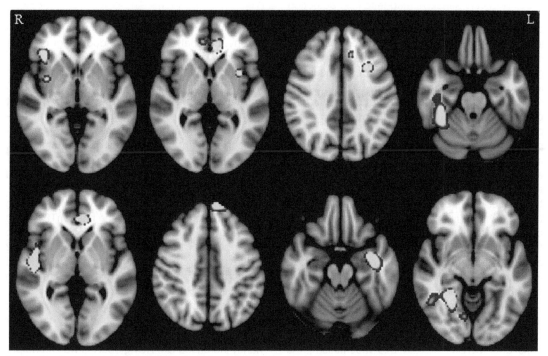

Fig. 5. Single subject–based analysis showing statistically abnormal MEG slow-wave sources in 8 representative mTBI cases (MNI-152 Atlas Coordinates).

Signal Processing, Forward Modeling, MEG Inverse Source Imaging, and Coherence Analysis," in this issue and Ref.[76]). Compared with controls, mTBI participants demonstrated striking gamma-band hyperactivity, mainly in (1) prefrontal areas, including bilateral lateral-FP (Brodmann area or BA 10) and right pars opercularis (BA 44)/pars triangularis (BA 45) of the inferior frontal gyrus; (2) bilateral supplementary motor area (medial BA 6) and right premotor cortex; (3) posterior parietal areas, including bilateral superior parietal lobule (BA 7), right supramarginal gurus (BA 40), and right angular gyrus (BA 39); (4) bilateral superior temporal gyri; (5) bilateral occipital areas, including cuneus, superior lateral occipital cortex (BA 19), and calcarine fissure (BA 17); and (6) right cerebellum (anterior lobe). Compared with the controls, mTBI participants also showed hypoactivity in ventromedial prefrontal cortex (vmPFC), midline anterior cingulate cortex, and the midbrain.[46]

Across groups, greater gamma activity correlated with poorer performances on tests of executive functioning and visuospatial processing. Many neurocognitive associations, however, were partly driven by the higher incidence of mTBI participants with both higher gamma activity and poorer cognition, suggesting that expansive upregulation of gamma has negative repercussions for cognition,

particularly in mTBI.[46] This human study is the first to demonstrate abnormal resting-state gamma activity in mTBI. These novel findings suggest the possibility that abnormal gamma activities may be a proxy for GABA-ergic interneuron dysfunction and a promising neuroimaging marker of insidious mild head injuries.[46]

MAGNETOENCEPHALOGRAPHY ABERRANT FUNCTIONAL CONNECTIVITY IN MILD TRAUMATIC BRAIN INJURY

As mentioned previously, a leading model of TBI, the DAI model, maintains that injury in WM tracts is a major contributor to the PCS and cognitive deficits in mTBI patients.[56] One expected consequence of reduced FA in WM is the disruption of neuronal communication between GM areas, which may lead to decreased FC with other brain regions, especially if axonal damage is substantial. For example, FA is consistently reduced in the WM of patients with Alzheimer disease[96–98] and schizophrenia.[99–101] Similarly, functional magnetic resonance (fMR) imaging studies report reduced FC among GM areas in both disorders.[102–105] However, decreased FC has not been found consistently in mTBI patients, suggesting that other mechanisms may also be at play (see review and references cited in Ref.[45]).

Another leading model for TBI is the glutamate-based overexcitation and GABA-ergic disinhibition injury model, which emphasizes injuries in GM neurons.[106–109] By this model, injury to the brain causes glutamate excitotoxicity in pyramidal neurons, leading to injury and death of GABA-ergic interneurons. The dysfunctional GABA-ergic interneurons create disinhibition in pyramidal neurons, which produces overexcitation. A similar mechanism is posited for posttraumatic epilepsy (see references in Ref.[110]), for which increased global FC is well established.[111] Thus, in contrast to the DAI model, the glutamate overexcitation and GABA disinhibition model posit aberrant GABA intraneuron functioning, which diminishes the inhibitory influence on pyramidal neurons, thereby causing increased firing and facilitation of network connections that are normally inhibited. This process could lead to increases in FC between the injured GM area and other regions of the brain.

Another mechanism that also predicts increases in FC is the functional reorganization model through compensation or rerouting of functional connections after mTBI.[112–116] In this mechanism, the areas showing the increases in FC are not limited to injured GM areas; noninjured GM areas can be involved as well.[112,116] To facilitate functional reorganization, reduced inhibition and increased excitation are also needed between GM brain regions, similar to the glutamate overexcitation GABA disinhibition injury model. However, the authors believe that the reduced inhibition in the functional reorganization model is not due to damages or death in GABA interneurons, but rather self-lifted inhibition in the GABA interneurons.

Measures of FC are of keen interest in mTBI because they are sensitive to disturbances in the communication among brain regions. In fMR imaging studies, both increased and decreased FC of the default mode network has been reported in blunt mTBI (see references cited in Ref.[45]), whereas a study using MEG found decreased FC of frontal and parietal-temporal-occipital regions in a mixed sample of mild, moderate, and severe TBI.[52] However, few studies have examined FC disturbances in blast mTBI.[117,118]

In a recent study by Huang and colleagues,[45] the regional patterns of aberrant whole-brain FC in blast mTBI patients were identified using resting-state MEG. Study participants included 26 active-duty service members or veterans who had blast mTBI with persistent PCS and 22 healthy control active-duty service members or veterans. MEG source imaging and source time courses were obtained using Fast-VESTAL. The source time courses from GM regions of interest (ROIs) were then used to compute ROI to whole-brain

(ROI-global) FC for 2 different measures: (1) time-lagged cross-correlation and (2) phase-lock synchrony. FC analyses were conducted for different frequency bands.

Compared with the controls, participants with blast mTBI showed increased GM ROI-global FC in beta-, gamma-, and low-frequency bands, but not in the alpha-band. Sources of abnormal increases in FC were from the following: (1) prefrontal cortex (right ventromedial prefrontal cortex, right rostral anterior cingulate cortex), left ventrolateral prefrontal cortex and DLPFC; (2) medial temporal lobe (bilateral parahippocampal gyri, hippocampi, and amygdala); and (3) right putamen and cerebellum. In contrast, the blast mTBI group also showed decreased FC of the right FP. Group differences were highly consistent for the 2 different FC measures. In addition, FC of the left ventrolateral prefrontal cortex correlated with cognitive functioning in mTBI participants.[45]

Overall, using 2 different types of FC measures (ie, time-lagged cross-correlation and phase-lock synchrony) to examine FC in blast TBI, predominantly increased GM ROI-global FC was found primarily in beta-, but also in gamma-, and low-frequency bands. The abnormal increases in FC were mainly from prefrontal and medial temporal lobe areas. In contrast, decreases in FC of the right FP were also observed in blast mTBI. Tests of group differences were highly consistent for the 2 different FC measures. Although the decreases in FC may be associated with DAI in WM tracts, the overwhelming findings of increased FC are compatible with glutamate-based overexcitation and GABA-ergic disinhibition of injured GM tissue.

EVENT-RELATED MAGNETIC FIELDS

As mentioned above, there have been some studies of MEG oscillatory activity in mTBI during task performance.[89,91] Another potentially useful approach to the study of information processing in TBI is to examine event-related magnetic fields. Event-related magnetic activity can be extracted from the MEG background through signal averaging techniques identical to those used for the extraction of event-related/evoked-response potentials (ERPs) in the EEG. Briefly, windows of spontaneous activity time locked to an event (ie, a stimulus presentation or a behavioral response) are averaged. Event-related responses are potentially of high utility for tracking in both space and time the patterns of brain activation associated with specific sensory, motor, and cognitive processes. ERPs (especially with respect to the P300 complex) have been used extensively to evaluate the information processing in head trauma, with data showing alterations in mTBI, at least at the group level.[119–121] To date, there has been surprisingly limited work exploring magnetic evoked fields in TBI. Much of the research has been performed by Taylor, Pang and colleagues,[122] who have used several different experimental paradigms, including those exploring intra-extradimensional set shifting and working memory.[123] There has also been a study by another group, this one using the Attention Network Test to examine cue-evoked P300m activity, contingent magnetic variation, and a target evoked P300m.[124] At the group level, each of these studies has shown decreased and sometimes delayed activation profiles for mTBI patients. It remains to be determined if findings are robust enough for identifying mTBI at the individual subject level.

Recently, some preliminary data have emerged to suggest that certain evoked field findings may be used for identifying individual subjects with chronic PCS after mTBI. In the MEG, it was previously reported by Iwasaki and colleagues[125] that median nerve somatosensory evoked fields were very abnormal in comatose survivors of severe TBI, especially with respect to the N30m component. Lewine and colleagues (2020, in preparation) have recently examined this situation in more than 100 mTBI patients and found that there is a subset of about 30% who have markedly attenuated or delayed N30m responses, as shown in **Fig. 6**. Although the sensitivity of the finding in mTBI is relatively low, specificity appears to be high with respect to both neurotypical control subjects and patients with a wide range of other conditions, including PTSD, substance abuse, major depressive disorder, and learning disability, all with an incidence rate for the observation of less than 5%. To date, the only other conditions whereby the rate of N30m abnormality has been seen to exceed 15% are rolandic epilepsies or cases whereby tumors compress primary somatosensory or motor regions. At present, it is thought that the M30m abnormality in mTBI reflects a general and perhaps widespread disruption of cortical inhibitory mechanisms, most easily indexed through the median nerve-evoked response.

Another evoked response of emerging interest in mTBI relates to auditory sensory gating. In a small EEG study, using a paired-click paradigm, Arciniegas and colleagues[126] found that subjects with mTBI failed to show normal sensory gating. Briefly, when 2 clicks are presented in rapid succession to neurotypical control subjects (with a 500-millisecond intertone interval, and a 2-second-long interstimulus interval between successive pairs), P50, N100, and P200 response components for the second tone are markedly attenuated/gated (at about 30%) relative to the response components to the first tone in the pair. In contrast, subjects with mTBI generally show gating ratios of greater than 50%. That is, they fail to gate.

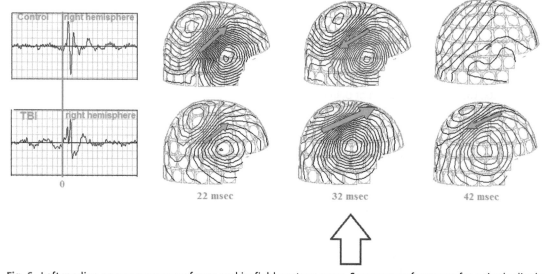

22 msec   32 msec   42 msec

Fig. 6. Left median nerve source waveforms and isofield contour maps. Source waveforms are for a single dipole fit over a time window from 15 to 45 milliseconds. Data were filtered at 10 to 150 Hz and baseline corrected. Each tick on the horizontal axis is 20 milliseconds. For the neurotypical control subjects, there is a strong M30m response with a 180° reversal in the direction of current flow between 22 and 32 milliseconds (P20m and N30m). In contrast, for the mTBI subject, current flow at 32 milliseconds (time marked by red arrow) is still pointing anteriorly, with posterior current flow delayed to 42 milliseconds.

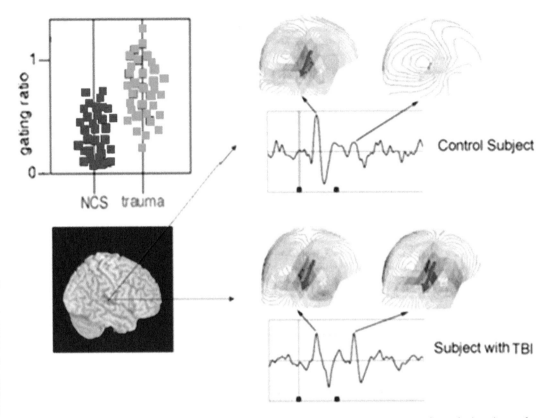

Fig. 7. N100m auditory sensory gating is impaired in subjects with mTBI. As shown in the right-hand waveforms and iso-field contour maps, the response to the second of two identical paired tones (indicated by the black boxes on the timeline) is markedly attenuated for the control subject (*top*), but not the subject with TBI (*bottom*). The gating ratio refers to the magnitude of the second response relative to the first response. The control subject shows a low gating ratio, an index of good sensory gating. The TBI subject shows a high gating ratio, an indication of failed sensory gating. The upper left hand panel shows the gating ratio for a group of Normal Control Subjects (NCS) and patients with head trauma.

Lewine and colleagues (2020, in preparation) have recently adapted this general approach for use in MEG, with the presentation of paired tones with an intertone interval of 300 milliseconds. In a study of 35 neurotypical control subjects and 35 patients with chronic PCS following an mTBI, it was found that N100m gating was significantly reduced in the mTBI group ($P<.005$; **Fig. 7**). When setting a gating ratio at a threshold of greater than 50% for at least 1 hemisphere, individual mTBI and control subjects could be distinguished with 74% accuracy. Like the somatosensory response discussed above, the gating abnormality is fairly specific to TBI. Subjects with PTSD, depression, or anxiety in the absence of TBI rarely show gating ratios greater than 50%. Even patients with schizophrenia (where gating issues were first described) only rarely show gating ratios >50%.[127] Given this, evaluation of auditory sensory gating may be of significant utility in the differential evaluation of patients with mTBI.

SUMMARY

The peer-reviewed scientific literature is increasingly demonstrating that MEG has much to offer in the evaluation of patients with mTBI. Importantly, presented methods for the evaluation of certain evoked responses and abnormal low-frequency magnetic activity and abnormal high-frequency magnetic activity are applicable at the single-subject level. To date, analyses of slow-wave activity are the most viable, with a clear neurobiological foundation and convergent data across approaches and multiple evaluation sites. Indeed, MEG slow-wave analyses are seeing increasing use in clinical, research, and forensic settings. At present, MEG is not intended for use as a stand-alone diagnostic test for mTBI, but when MEG evaluation is included in a multifactorial evaluation of the potential neurobiological consequences of head trauma, it can provide for sensitive and objective documentation of brain injury and pathophysiology, with information from patient history and other tests providing differential etiologic conclusions.

MAGNETOENCEPHALOGRAPHY SOURCE IMAGING FOR POSTTRAUMATIC STRESS DISORDER

PTSD is another leading health issue in active-duty military personnel, veterans, and the general public. Individuals exposed to a traumatic event may develop PTSD with debilitating posttraumatic stress symptoms, including intrusive memories, avoidance behavior, emotional numbing, and hyperarousal.[128] PTSD is a major health concern that affects approximately 7.7% of Americans[129,130] and is particularly prevalent among military service members who have served in combat.[131,132] The combat veterans returning from the wars in Iraq and Afghanistan have shown elevated rates of PTSD.[133–135] Indirect functional neuroimaging studies using PET or fMR imaging with fear-related stimuli support a PTSD neurocircuitry model that includes amygdala, hippocampus, and vmPFC. However, it is not clear if this model can fully account for PTSD abnormalities detected directly by electromagnetic-based source imaging techniques in resting state.[136]

Electromagnetic measures such as MEG provide direct measurements of neuronal activity in PTSD. Using an MEG sensor-space synchronous neural interactions analysis, Georgopoulos and colleagues[137] and Engdahl and colleagues[138] correctly classified individuals with PTSD and healthy control subjects with greater than 90% overall accuracy of classification. They also found differences in MEG communication measures between temporal and parietal and/or parietooccipital right hemispheric areas with other brain areas in PTSD.

MEG source imaging has been used in studying the PTSD neurocircuitry. The study by Huang and colleagues[139] examined resting-state MEG signals in 25 active-duty service members and veterans with PTSD and 30 healthy volunteers. In contrast to the healthy volunteers, individuals with PTSD showed the following: (1) hyperactivity from amygdala, hippocampus, posterolateral OFC, dorsomedial prefrontal cortex, and insular cortex in high-frequency (ie, beta-, gamma-, and high gamma-) bands; (2) hypoactivity from vmPFC, FP, and dLPFC in high-frequency bands; (3) extensive hypoactivity from dLPFC, FP, anterior temporal

lobes, precuneus cortex, and sensorimotor cortex in alpha- and low-frequency bands; (4) in individuals with PTSD, MEG activity in the left amygdala, and posterolateral OFC correlated positively with PTSD symptom scores, whereas MEG activity in vmPFC and precuneus correlated negatively with symptom score. That study showed that MEG source imaging technique revealed new abnormalities in the resting-state electromagnetic signals from the PTSD neurocircuitry. In particular, posterolateral OFC and precuneus may play important roles in the PTSD neurocircuitry model.

ACKNOWLEDGMENTS

This work was supported in part by Merit Review Grants from the U.S. Department of Veterans Affairs to M.X.H and R.R.L (I01-CX002035-01, NURC-007-19S, I01-CX000499, MHBA-010-14F, I01-RX001988, B1988-I, NURC-022-10F, NEUC-044-06S), and a grant from the Illinois Department of Veterans Affairs to JDL (Alexian-01).

DISCLOSURE

The authors have nothing to disclose.

REFERENCES

1. Centers for Disease Control and Prevention, National Center for Injury Prevention and Control. Report to Congress on mild traumatic brain injury in the United States: steps to prevent a serious public health problem. Atlanta (GA): Centers for Disease Control and Prevention; 2003.
2. Department of Health and Human Services, Interagency report of the head injury task force, Washington, DC: 1989.
3. Pope AM, Taylor AR. Disability in America: toward a national agenda for prevention. Washington, DC: National Academic Press; 1991.
4. Stachniak J, Layton AJ. Closed head injury and the treatment of sequelae after a motor vehicle accident. J Clin Anesth 1994;6:437–49.
5. Fedele B, Williams G, McKenzie D, et al. Subacute sleep disturbance in moderate to severe traumatic brain injury: a systematic review. Brain Inj 2019;27:1–12.
6. Hoofien D, Gilboa A, Vakil E, et al. Traumatic brain injury (TBI) 10-20 years later: a comprehensive study of psychiatric symptomatology, cognitive abilities and psychosocial functioning. Brain Inj 2001;15:189–209.
7. Kwentus JA, Hart RP, Peck ET, et al. Psychiatric complications of closed head trauma. Psychosomatics 1985;26:8–15.
8. Ryttersgaard TO, Johnsen SP, Riis JO, et al. Prevalence of depression after moderate to severe

traumatic brain injury among adolescents and young adults: a systematic review. Scand J Psychol 2019;61(2):297–306.

9. Ruff RM, Buchsbaum MD, Troster AL, et al. Computerized tomography, neuropsychology, and positron emission tomography in the evaluation of head injury. Neuropsychiatry Neuropsychol Behav Neurol 1989;2:103–23.

10. Vakil E, Greenstein Y, Weiss I, et al. The effects of moderate-to-severe traumatic brain injury on episodic memory: a meta-analysis. Neuropsychol Rev 2019;29:270–87.

11. Barth J, Macciocchi S, Giordani B. Neuropsychological sequelae of minor head injury. Neurosurgery 1983;13:520–37.

12. Bigler ED. Neuropsychology and clinical neuroscience of persistent post-concussive syndrome. J Int Neuropsychol Soc 2008;14:1–22.

13. Binder LM. A review of mild head trauma. Part II: clinical implications. J Clin Exp Neuropsychol 1997;19:432–57.

14. Bohnen NI, Jolles J, Twijnstra A, et al. Late neurobehavioral symptoms after mild head injury. Brain Inj 1995;9:27–33.

15. Boyle E, Cancelliere C, Hartvigsen J, et al. Systematic review of prognosis after mild traumatic brain injury in the military: results of the International Collaboration on Mild Traumatic Brain Injury Prognosis. Arch Phys Med Rehabil 2014;95:S230–7.

16. McAllister T, McCrea M. Long-term cognitive and neuropsychiatric consequences of repetitive concussion and head-impact exposure. J Athl Train 2017;52:309–17.

17. McInnes K, Friesen CL, MacKenzie DE, et al. Mild traumatic brain injury (mTBI) and chronic cognitive impairment: a scoping review. PLoS One 2017;12: e0174847.

18. Voller B, Benke T, Benedetto K, et al. Neuropsychological, MRI and EEG findings after very mild traumatic brain injury. Brain Inj 1999;13:821–7.

19. Kraus JF, McArthur DL, Silberman TA. Epidemiology of mild brain injury. Semin Neurol 1994;14: 1–7.

20. Alosco ML, Stern RA. The long-term consequences of repetitive head impacts: chronic traumatic encephalopathy. Handb Clin Neurol 2019;167: 337–55.

21. Rabadi MH, Jordan BD. The cumulative effect of repetitive concussion in sports. Clin J Sport Med 2001;11(3):194–8.

22. Barnes DE, Byers AL, Gardner RC, et al. Association of mild traumatic brain injury with and without loss of consciousness with dementia in US military veterans. JAMA Neurol 2018;75(9):1055–61.

23. Guo Z, Cupples LA, Kurz A, et al. Head injury and risk of AD in the MIRAGE study. Neurology 2000; 54:1316–23.

24. LoBue CD, Denney D, Hynan LS, et al. Self-reported traumatic brain injury and mild cognitive impairment: increased risk and earlier age of diagnosis. J Alzheimers Dis 2016;51(3):727–36.

25. Mayeux R, Otiman R, Maestre G, et al. Synergistic effects of traumatic head injury and apolipoprotein-epsilon 4 in subjects with Alzheimer's disease. Neurology 1995;45:555–7.

26. Nordstrom P, Michaelsson K, Gustafson Y, et al. Traumatic brain injury and young onset dementia: a nationwide cohort study. Ann Neurol 2014;75(3): 374–81.

27. Plassman BL, Havlik RJ, Steffens DC, et al. Documented head injury in early adulthood and risk of Alzheimer's disease and other dementias. Neurology 2000;55:1158–66.

28. Massel BE, DeWitt DS. Traumatic brain injury: a disease process, not an event. J Neurotrauma 2010;27:1529–40.

29. Wener C, Engelhard K. Pathophysiology of traumatic brain injury. Br J Anaesth 2007;99:4–9.

30. Jeter CB, Hergenroeder GW, Hylin MJ, et al. Biomarkers for the diagnosis and prognosis of mild traumatic brain injury/concussion. J Neurotrauma 2013;30:657–70.

31. Johnston KM, Ptito A, Chankowsky J, et al. New frontiers in diagnostic imaging in concussive head injury. Clin J Sport Med 2001;11:166–75.

32. van der Naalt J, Hew JM, van Zomeren AH, et al. Computed tomography and magnetic resonance imaging in mild to moderate head injury: early and late imaging related to outcome. Ann Neurol 1999;46:70–8.

33. Leininger BE, Gramling SE, Farrell ED, et al. Neuropsychological deficits in symptomatic minor head injury subjects after concussion and mild concussion. J Neurol Neurosurg Psychiatry 1990;53:293–6.

34. Margulies S. The postconcussion syndrome after mild head trauma: is brain damage overdiagnosed? Part 1. J Clin Neurosci 2000;7:400–8.

35. Miller H. Accident neurosis. Br Med J 1961;1: 919–25.

36. Bigler ED, Snyder JL. Neuropsychological outcome and quantitative neuroimaging in mild head injury. Arch Clin Neuropsychol 1995;10:159–74.

37. Mayer AR, Ling J, Mannell MV, et al. A prospective diffusion tensor imaging study in mild traumatic brain injury. Neurology 2010;74(8):643–50.

38. Ross DE, Ochs AL, Seabaugh JM, et al. Man versus machine: comparison of radiologists' interpretations and NeuroQuant® volumetric analyses of brain MRIs in patients with traumatic brain injury. J Neuropsychiatry Clin Neurosci 2013;25(1):32–9.

39. Wallace EJ, Mathias JL, Ward L. Diffusion tensor imaging changes following mild, moderate and severe adult traumatic brain injury: a meta-analysis. Brain Imaging Behav 2018;12(6):1607–21.

40. Abdel-Dayem HM, Abu-Judeh H, Kumar M, et al. SPECT brain perfusion abnormalities in mild or moderate traumatic brain injury. Clin Nucl Med 1998;23:309–17.

41. Chen S, Kareken D, Fastenau P, et al. A study of persistent postconcussion symptoms in mild head trauma using positron emission tomography. J Neurol Neurosurg Psychiatry 2003;74:326–32.

42. Raji CA, Henderson TA. PET and single-photon emission computed tomography in brain concussion. Neuroimaging Clin N Am 2018;28(1):67–82.

43. Raji CA, Tarzwell R, Pavel D, et al. Clinical utility of SPECT neuroimaging in the diagnosis and treatment of traumatic brain injury: a systematic review. PLoS One 2014;9(3):e91088.

44. Hanley D, Prichep LS, Badjatia N, et al. A brain electrical activity electroencephalographic-based biomarker of functional impairment in traumatic brain injury: a multi-site validation trial. J Neurotrauma 2018;35(1):41–7.

45. Huang M-X, Harrington DL, Robb Swan A, et al. Resting-state magnetoencephalography reveals different patterns of aberrant functional connectivity in combat-related mild traumatic brain injury. J Neurotrauma 2017;34:1412–26.

46. Huang M-X, Huang CW, Harrington DL, et al. Marked increases in resting-state MEG gamma-band activity in combat-related mild traumatic brain Injury. Cereb Cortex 2019. https://doi.org/10.1093/cercor/bhz087.

47. Huang M-X, Nichols S, Baker DG, et al. Single-subject-based whole-brain MEG slow-wave imaging approach for detecting abnormality in patients with mild traumatic brain injury. Neuroimage Clin 2014;5:109–19.

48. Huang M-X, Nichols S, Robb A, et al. An automatic MEG low-frequency source imaging approach for detecting injuries in mild and moderate TBI patients with blast and non-blast causes. NeuroImage 2012;61:1067–82.

49. Lew HL, Lee EH, Pan SS, et al. Electrophysiologic abnormalities of auditory and visual information processing in patients with traumatic brain injury. Am J Phys Med Rehabil 2004;83(6):428–33.

50. Lewine JD, Davis JT, Bigler ED, et al. Objective documentation of traumatic brain injury subsequent to mild head trauma: multimodal brain imaging with MEG, SPECT, and MRI. J Head Trauma Rehabil 2007;22:141–55.

51. Lewine JD, Orrison WW, Sloan JH, et al. Neuromagnetic assessment of pathophysiological brain activity induced by minor head trauma. AJNR Am J Neuroradiol 1999;20:857–66.

52. Tarapore PE, Findlay AM, Lahue SC, et al. Resting state magnetoencephalography functional connectivity in traumatic brain injury. J Neurosurg 2013;118:1306–16.

53. Thatcher RW, North DM, Curtin RT, et al. An EEG severity index of traumatic brain injury. J Neuropsychiatry Clin Neurosci 2001;13(1):77–87.

54. Garman RH, Jenkins LW, Switzer RC III, et al. Blast exposure in rats with body shielding is characterized primarily by diffuse axonal injury. J Neurotrauma 2011;28:947–59.

55. Asken BM, DeKosky ST, Clugston JR, et al. Diffusion tensor imaging (DTI) findings in adult civilian, military, and sport-related mild traumatic brain injury (mTBI): a systematic critical review. Brain Imaging Behav 2018;12:585–612.

56. Hannawi Y, Stevens RD. Mapping the connectome following traumatic brain injury. Curr Neurol Neurosci Rep 2016;16:44.

57. Lewine JD. Brain imaging in mild traumatic brain injury. In: Zollman FS, editor. Manual of traumatic brain injury management. 2nd edition. New York: Demos Medical; 2016. p. 82–90.

58. Davenport ND, Lim KO, Armstrong MT, et al. Diffuse and spatially variable white matter disruptions are associated with blast-related mild traumatic brain injury. Neuroimage 2012;59:2017–24.

59. Mac Donald CL, Johnson AM, Cooper D, et al. Detection of blast-related traumatic brain injury in U.S. military personnel. N Engl J Med 2011;364:2091–100.

60. Shenton ME, Hamoda HM, Schneiderman JS, et al. A review of magnetic resonance imaging and diffusion tensor imaging findings in mild traumatic brain injury. Brain Imaging Behav 2012;6:137–92.

61. Shizukuishi T, Abe O, Aoki S. Diffusion tensor imaging analysis in psychiatric disorders. Magn Reson Med Sci 2013;12(3):153–9.

62. Tae WS, Ham BJ, Pyun SB, et al. Current clinical applications of diffusion-tensor imaging in neurological disorders. J Clin Neurol 2018;14(2):129–40.

63. Vascak M, Jin X, Jacobs KM, et al. Mild traumatic brain injury induces structural and functional disconnection of local neocortical inhibitory networks via parvalbumin interneuron diffuse axonal injury. Cereb Cortex 2018;28:1625–44.

64. Kobeissy FH, editor. Brain neurotrauma: molecular, neuropsychological, and rehabilitation aspects. Boca Raton (FL): CRC Press/Taylor & Francis; 2015.

65. Ball GJ, Gloor P, Schaul N. The cortical electromicrophysiology of pathological delta waves in the electroencephalogram of cats. Electroencephalogr Clin Neurophysiol 1977;43:346–61.

66. Gloor P, Ball G, Schaul N. Brain lesions that produce delta waves in the EEG. Neurology 1977;27:326–33.

67. Schaul N. The fundamental neural mechanisms of electroencephalography. Electroencephalogr Clin Neurophysiol 1998;106:101–7.

68. Schaul N, Gloor P, Ball G, et al. The electromicrophysiology of delta waves induced by systemic atropine. Brain Res 1978;143:475–86.

69. Fauught E. Current role of electroencephalography in cerebra ischemia. Stroke 1993;24(4):609–13.

70. Wolpow ER. Focal rhythmic EEG slowing with temporal lobe tumors. Report of six cases. Confin Neurol 1973;35(4):193–201.

71. deJongh A, de Munck JC, Baayen JC, et al. The localization of spontaneous brain activity: first results in patients with cerebral tumors. Clin Neurophysiol 2001;112:378–85.

72. Vieth JB, Kober H, Grummich P. Sources of spontaneous slow wave associated with brain lesions localized by using the MEG. Brain Topogr 1996;8:215–22.

73. Lewine JD, Orrison WW. Spike and slow wave localization by magnetoencephalography. Neuroimaging Clin N Am 1995;5(4):575–96.

74. Lewine JD, Fisch BJ, Bangera N. Fundamentals of magnetoencephalography. In: Nofzinger E, Maquet P, Thorpy M, editors. Neuroimaging of sleep and sleep disorders. Cambridge (England): Cambridge University Press; 2013. p. 62–71.

75. Robb Swan A, Nichols S, Drake A, et al. Magnetoencephalography slow-wave detection in patients with mild traumatic brain injury and ongoing symptoms correlated with long-term neuropsychological outcome. J Neurotrauma 2015;32:1510–21.

76. Huang M-X, Huang CW, Robb A, et al. MEG source imaging method using fast L1 minimum-norm and its applications to signals with brain noise and human resting-state source amplitude images. NeuroImage 2014;84:585–604.

77. Hsieh T-H, Lee HHC, Hameed MQ, et al. Trajectory of parvalbumin cell impairment and loss of cortical inhibition in traumatic brain injury. Cereb Cortex 2017;27:5509–24.

78. Carlén M, Meletis K, Siegle JH, et al. A critical role for NMDA receptors in parvalbumin interneurons for gamma rhythm induction and behavior. Mol Psychiatry 2012;17:537–48.

79. Jones RS, Bühl EH. Basket-like interneurones in layer II of the entorhinal cortex exhibit a powerful NMDA-mediated synaptic excitation. Neurosci Lett 1993;149:35–9.

80. Cardin JA, Carlén M, Meletis K, et al. Driving fast-spiking cells induces gamma rhythm and controls sensory responses. Nature 2009;459:663–7.

81. Fries P. Neuronal gamma-band synchronization as a fundamental process in cortical computation. Annu Rev Neurosci 2009;32:209–24.

82. Sohal VS, Zhang F, Yizhar O, et al. Parvalbumin neurons and gamma rhythms enhance cortical circuit performance. Nature 2009;459:698–702.

83. Traub RD, Whittington MA, Stanford IM, et al. A mechanism for generation of long-range synchronous fast oscillations in the cortex. Nature 1996;383:621–4.

84. Cho KKA, Hoch R, Lee AT, et al. Gamma rhythms link prefrontal interneuron dysfunction with cognitive inflexibility in Dlx5/6(+/-) mice. Neuron 2015;85:1332–43.

85. Kalemaki K, Konstantoudaki X, Tivodar S, et al. Mice with decreased number of interneurons exhibit aberrant spontaneous and oscillatory activity in the cortex. Front Neural Circuits 2018;12:96.

86. Del Pino I, García-Frigola C, Dehorter N, et al. Erbb4 deletion from fast-spiking interneurons causes schizophrenia-like phenotypes. Neuron 2013;79:1152–68.

87. Korotkova T, Fuchs EC, Ponomarenko A, et al. NMDA receptor ablation on parvalbumin-positive interneurons impairs hippocampal synchrony, spatial representations, and working memory. Neuron 2010;68:557–69.

88. Bartos M, Vida I, Jonas P. Synaptic mechanisms of synchronized gamma oscillations in inhibitory interneuron networks. Nat Rev Neurosci 2007;8:45–56.

89. Huang M-X, Nichols S, Robb-Swan A, et al. MEG working memory n-back task reveals functional deficits in combat-related mild traumatic brain injury. Cereb Cortex 2019;29:1953–68.

90. Bailey NW, Rogasch NC, Hoy KE, et al. Increased gamma connectivity during working memory retention following traumatic brain injury. Brain Inj 2017;31:379–89.

91. Slewa-Younan S, Green AM, Baguley IJ, et al. Is "gamma" (40 Hz) synchronous activity disturbed in patients with traumatic brain injury? Clin Neurophysiol 2002;113:1640–6.

92. Spooner RK, Wiesman AI, Mills MS, et al. Aberrant oscillatory dynamics during somatosensory processing in HIV-infected adults. Neuroimage Clin 2018;20:85–91.

93. Kwon JS, O'Donnell BF, Wallenstein GV, et al. Gamma frequency-range abnormalities to auditory stimulation in schizophrenia. Arch Gen Psychiatry 1999;56:1001–5.

94. Popov T, Jordanov T, Weisz N, et al. Evoked and induced oscillatory activity contributes to abnormal auditory sensory gating in schizophrenia. NeuroImage 2011;56:307–14.

95. Buzhdygan T, Lisinicchia J, Patel V, et al. Neuropsychological, neurovirological and neuroimmune aspects of abnormal GABAergic transmission in HIV infection. J Neuroimmune Pharmacol 2016;11:279–93.

96. Douaud G, Menke RA, Gass A, et al. Brain microstructure reveals early abnormalities more than two years prior to clinical progression from mild cognitive impairment to Alzheimer's disease. J Neurosci 2013;33:2147–55.

97. Kantarci K. Fractional anisotropy of the fornix and hippocampal atrophy in Alzheimer's disease. Front Aging Neurosci 2014;6:316.

98. Mielke MM, Okonkwo OC, Oishi K, et al. Fornix integrity and hippocampal volume predict memory

decline and progression to Alzheimer's disease. Alzheimers Dement 2012;8:105–13.

99. Ellison-Wright I, Bullmore E. Meta-analysis of diffusion tensor imaging studies in schizophrenia. Schizophr Res 2009;108:3–10.

100. Fitzsimmons J, Kubicki M, Shenton ME. Review of functional and anatomical brain connectivity findings in schizophrenia. Curr Opin Psychiatry 2013; 26:172–87.

101. Tamnes CK, Agartz I. White matter microstructure in early-onset schizophrenia: a systematic review of diffusion tensor imaging studies. J Am Acad Child Adolesc Psychiatry 2016;55:269–79.

102. Chen Y, Yan H, Han Z, et al. Functional activity and connectivity differences of five resting-state networks in patients with alzheimer's disease or mild cognitive impairment. Curr Alzheimer Res 2016; 13:234–42.

103. Greicius MD, Srivastava G, Reiss AL, et al. Default-mode network activity distinguishes Alzheimer's disease from healthy aging: evidence from functional MRI. Proc Natl Acad Sci U S A 2004;101: 4637–42.

104. Schilbach L, Hoffstaedter F, Muller V, et al. Trans-diagnostic commonalities and differences in resting state functional connectivity of the default mode network in schizophrenia and major depression. Neuroimage Clin 2016;10:326–35.

105. Sorg C, Riedl V, Muhlau M, et al. Selective changes of resting-state networks in individuals at risk for Alzheimer's disease. Proc Natl Acad Sci U S A 2007;104:18760–5.

106. Almeida-Suhett CP, Prager EM, Pidoplichko V, et al. Reduced GABAergic inhibition in the basolateral amygdala and the development of anxiety-like behaviors after mild traumatic brain injury. PLoS One 2014;9:e102627.

107. Cantu D, Walker K, Andresen L, et al. Traumatic brain injury increases cortical glutamate network activity by compromising GABAergic control. Cereb Cortex 2015;25:2306–20.

108. Giza CC, Hovda DA. The new neurometabolic cascade of concussion. Neurosurgery 2014; 75(Suppl 4):S24–33.

109. Guerriero RM, Giza CC, Rotenberg A. Glutamate and GABA imbalance following traumatic brain injury. Curr Neurol Neurosci Rep 2015;15:27.

110. Prince DA, Parada I, Scalise K, et al. Epilepsy following cortical injury: cellular and molecular mechanisms as targets for potential prophylaxis. Epilepsia 2009;50(Suppl 2):30–40.

111. Song J, Nair VA, Gaggl W, et al. Disrupted brain functional organization in epilepsy revealed by graph theory analysis. Brain Connect 2015;5:276–83.

112. Mayer AR, Mannell MV, Ling J, et al. Functional connectivity in mild traumatic brain injury. Hum Brain Mapp 2011;32:1825–35.

113. Nathan DE, Oakes TR, Yeh PH, et al. Exploring variations in functional connectivity of the resting state default mode network in mild traumatic brain injury. Brain Connect 2015;5:102–14.

114. Sours C, Chen H, Roys S, et al. Investigation of multiple frequency ranges using discrete wavelet decomposition of resting-state functional connectivity in mild traumatic brain injury patients. Brain Connect 2015;5:442–50.

115. Sours C, George EO, Zhuo J, et al. Hyper-connectivity of the thalamus during early stages following mild traumatic brain injury. Brain Imaging Behav 2015;9:550–63.

116. Tang CY, Eaves E, ms-O'Connor K, et al. Diffuse disconnectivity in TBI: a resting state fMRI and DTI study. Transl Neurosci 2012;3:9–14.

117. Han K, Mac Donald CL, Johnson AM, et al. Disrupted modular organization of resting-state cortical functional connectivity in U.S. military personnel following concussive "mild" blast-related traumatic brain injury. Neuroimage 2014; 84:76–96.

118. Robinson ME, Lindemer ER, Fonda JR, et al. Close-range blast exposure is associated with altered functional connectivity in veterans independent of concussion symptoms at time of exposure. Hum Brain Mapp 2015;36:911–22.

119. Folmer RL, Billings CJ, Diedesch-Rouse AC, et al. Electrophysiological assessments of cognition and sensory processing in TBI: applications for diagnosis, prognosis, and rehabilitation. Int J Psychophysiol 2011;82(1):4–15.

120. Gilmore CS, Marquardt CA, Kang SS, et al. Reduced P3b brain response during sustained visual attention is associated with remote blast mTBI and current PTSD in U.S. military veterans. Behav Brain Res 2018;340:174–82.

121. Soldatovic-Stajic B, Misic-Pavkov G, Bozic K, et al. Neuropsychological and neurophysiological evaluation of cognitive deficits related to the severity of traumatic brain injury. Eur Rev Med Pharmacol Sci 2014;18(11):1632–7.

122. da Costa L, Robertson A, Bethune A, MacDonald MJ, et al. Delayed and disorganized brain activation detected with magnetoencephalography after mild traumatic brain injury. J Neurol Neurosurg Psychiatry 2015;86(9):1008–15.

123. Shah-Basak PP, Urbain C, Wong S, et al. Concussion alters the functional brain processes of visual attention and working memory. J Neurotrauma 2018;35(2):267–77.

124. Petley L, Bardoulle T, Chiasson D, et al. Attentional dysfunction and recovery in concussion: effects on the P300m and contingent magnetic variation. Brain Inj 2018;32(4):4640473.

125. Iwasaki M, Nakasato M, Kanno A, et al. Somatosensory evoked fields in comatose survivors after

severe traumatic brain injury. Clin Neurophysiol 2001;112:205–11.

126. Arciniegas D, Olincy A, Popkoff J, et al. Impaired auditory gating and P50 nonsuppression following traumatic brain injury. J Neuropsychiatry Clin Neurosci 2000;12(1):77–85.

127. Thoma RJ, Meier A, Houck J, et al. Auditory sensory gating during active auditory hallucinations. Schizophr Res 2017;188:125–31.

128. American Psychiatric Association. Practice guideline for the treatment of patients with acute stress disorder and PTSD. Arlington (VA): American Psychiatric Association Practice Guidelines; 2004.

129. Kessler RC, Berglund P, Demler O, et al. Lifetime prevalence and age-of-onset distributions of DSM-IV disorders in the National Comorbidity Survey Replication. Arch Gen Psychiatry 2005;62: 593–602.

130. Kessler RC, Sonnega A, Bromet E, et al. Posttraumatic stress disorder in the National Comorbidity Survey. Arch Gen Psychiatry 1995;52:1048–60.

131. Dohrenwend BP, Turner JB, Turse NA, et al. The psychological risks of Vietnam for U.S. veterans: a revisit with new data and methods. Science 2006;313:979–82.

132. Magruder KM, Yeager DE. The prevalence of PTSD across war eras and the effect of deployment on PTSD:a systematic review and meta-analysis. Psychiatr Ann 2009;39:778–88.

133. Hoge CW, Castro CA, Messer SC, et al. Combat duty in Iraq and Afghanistan, mental health

problems, and barriers to care. N Engl J Med 2004;351:13–22.

134. Smith TC, Ryan MA, Wingard DL, et al. New onset and persistent symptoms of post-traumatic stress disorder self reported after deployment and combat exposures: prospective population based US military cohort study. BMJ 2008;336:366–71.

135. Tanielian T, Jaycox LH. Invisible wounds of war: psychological and cognitive injuries, their consequences, and services to assist recovery. Santa Monica (CA): RAND Corporation; 2008.

136. Huang M, Risling M, Baker DG. The role of biomarkers and MEG-based imaging markers in the diagnosis of post-traumatic stress disorder and blast-induced mild traumatic brain injury. Psychoneuroendocrinology 2016;63:398–409.

137. Georgopoulos AP, Tan HR, Lewis SM, et al. The synchronous neural interactions test as a functional neuromarker for post-traumatic stress disorder (PTSD): a robust classification method based on the bootstrap. J Neural Eng 2010;7:16011.

138. Engdahl B, Leuthold AC, Tan H-R, et al. Post-traumatic stress disorder: a right temporal lobe syndrome? J Neural Eng 2010;7:066005.

139. Huang M-X, Yurgil KA, Robb A, et al. Voxel-wise resting-state MEG source magnitude imaging study reveals neurocircuitry abnormality in active-duty service members and veterans with PTSD. Neuroimage Clin 2014;5:408–19.

Magnetoencephalography Research in Pediatric Autism Spectrum Disorder

Heather L. Green, PhD[a],*, J. Christopher Edgar, PhD[a,b],
Junko Matsuzaki, PhD[a], Timothy P.L. Roberts, PhD[a,b]

KEYWORDS

- ASD • MEG • Biomarker • M50 • M100 • MMF • ERD

KEY POINTS

- MEG is not currently used clinically for diagnosis of ASD.
- Passive MEG paradigms are well suited for obtaining information on cortical function in children with ASD and thus have the potential for clinical use.
- Research has shown event-related and resting-state electrophysiological differences in individuals with ASD.
- Further research is needed to determine the diagnostic, prognostic, and therapeutic usefulness of MEG in this area.

INTRODUCTION

Over the last 25 years, there has been interest in understanding brain function in individuals with autism spectrum disorder (ASD). Autism was first described by Leo Kanner in 1943[1] and is characterized by deficits of social communication, interaction, and restricted and repetitive interests manifested in multiple situations and contexts.[2] In recent years, the prevalence of ASD has been on the increase, with current estimates of 1 in 40 children in the United States with autism.[3] As a result of the cognitive deficits common in ASD, many children with ASD require special education or therapeutic services. It is estimated that 89% of children with ASD receive special education services, with only 20% receiving services before the age of 2 years.[3] The societal and personal costs of ASD on affected individuals and families make elucidating the underlying causes of the disorder a top research priority.

A diagnosis of ASD is made via observation by trained clinicians. The median age of ASD

Disclaimer: Dr T.P.L. Roberts declares his position on the advisory boards of CTF MEG, Ricoh, Spago Nano Medical, and Prism Clinical Imaging, and consulting arrangements with Avexis Inc. and Acadia Pharmaceuticals. Dr T.P.L. Roberts and Dr J.C. Edgar also declare intellectual property relating to the potential use of electrophysiological markers for treatment planning in clinical ASD.
This article was supported in part by NIH grants R01DC008871 (to T.P.L. Roberts), R21NS106135 (to T.P.L. Roberts), R21MH109158 (to T.P.L. Roberts), R01MH107506 (to J.C. Edgar), R21MH098204 (to J.C. Edgar), R21NS090192 (to J.C. Edgar), NICHD grant R01HD093776 (to J.C. Edgar), and the Clinical Translational Core, Biostatistics & Bioinformatics Core and the Neuroimaging Core of the Intellectual and Developmental Disabilities Research Center funded by NICHD grant 5U54HD086984 (neuroimaging and neurocircuitry core director: TR; overall PI: M. Robinson, PhD). T.P.L. Roberts gratefully acknowledges the Oberkircher Family for the Oberkircher Family Chair in Pediatric Radiology at CHOP.
[a] Department of Radiology, Lurie Family Foundations MEG Imaging Center, The Children's Hospital of Philadelphia, 3401 Civic Center Boulevard, Philadelphia, PA 19104, USA; [b] Department of Radiology, Perelman School of Medicine, University of Pennsylvania, 3400 Civic Center Boulevard, Philadelphia, PA 19104, USA
* Corresponding author. Children's Hospital of Philadelphia, 3401 Civic Center Boulevard, Philadelphia, PA 19104, USA
E-mail address: greenhl@email.chop.edu

diagnosis in the United States is 4 years.[4] At present, there is no ASD brain imaging marker for clinical use. Individuals with ASD are not referred for clinical radiology examinations except in cases where there are comorbid medical concerns (eg, epilepsy, tuberous sclerosis). Neuroimaging, however, has often been proposed as a way to reduce diagnostic subjectivity as well as to identify at-risk infants who will go on to develop ASD.

Noninvasive, passive imaging techniques that do not require patient cooperation allow for easier assessment of difficult to assess populations (eg, infants, children, individuals with language or intellectual impairment). Magnetoencephalography (MEG) can be used in infants and young children and does not make any sound during measurement. MEG has the temporal resolution required to measure neural processing associated with incoming sensory information as well as for evaluating real-time cortical activity, such as resting-state brain activity. As detailed below, active areas of research seek neurophysiological diagnostic or prognostic measures of autism.

CANDIDATE BRAIN MARKERS OF AUTISM SPECTRUM DISORDER

MEG research in ASD is extensive, covering multiple sensory and cognitive modalities. Given space limitations, rather than provide an exhaustive review of all ASD MEG research, this article focuses on two areas of very active research: auditory processes and resting-state activity in ASD.

Numerous studies have revealed auditory processing and resting-state abnormalities in individuals with ASD.[5–17] Demonstrating these abnormalities at the single-subject level in children with ASD could lead to identifying neurophysiological "red flags" in infants and toddlers, long before clinical interviews identify children with ASD. Several candidate MEG "markers" are described.

M50 and M100

N100 and its magnetic equivalent N100m or M100, is a middle-latency auditory-evoked potential occurring approximately 100 ms after stimulus presentation. The auditory M100 response is regarded as an index of early sound perception and feature encoding, and is bilaterally generated in Heschl's gyrus and the planum temporale.[18,19] M100 latency decreases and amplitude increases as a function of age,[8,15,20,21] although in infants, toddlers, and young children M100 is not always observed.[8] By 10 to 12 years, adult-like M100 is observed in more than 80% of children.[8,22] M100 matures faster in the right hemisphere, with earlier latencies and larger amplitudes apparent at earlier time points in the right than in the left hemisphere.[8] M100 latency and amplitude are modulated by stimulus duration, intensity, or frequency with mid-frequency sounds (1–3 kHz) resulting in earlier M100 responses than lower frequency (100–200 Hz) sounds.[23,24] This M100 latency difference has been termed "dynamic range" and is approximately 10 to 15 ms in typically developing (TD) individuals.[23]

Although a small response in adults, the P50 or M50 is much more likely than the M100 to be observed in infants and young children, with a peak latency of 86 to 95 ms in 5 to 6 year olds.[25] MEG studies suggest that M50 is generated in the left and right superior temporal gyrus (STG).[26–31] Maturation of M50 occurs bilaterally, with both latency and amplitude decreasing with age.[21]

Several studies show later M50[8,16] and M100 latencies in individuals with ASD compared with TD controls, indicating delayed sound perception.[6,8,9,13,15,16,32] In a study of 25 children with ASD and 17 TD comparison children, Roberts and colleagues[15] found increased M100 latency in individuals with ASD in response to sinusoidal tones. The right hemisphere response to the 500 ms tone was a fair predictor of ASD (75% sensitivity, 81% specificity). These findings were replicated in a larger sample by Edgar and colleagues,[6] examining 52 children with ASD and 63 TD children aged 6 to 14 years. When a subset of children from these studies (ASD, 7; TD, 9; mean age 12.1 years) were recruited to a longitudinal study, the latency differences found at earlier time points were again observed 2 to 5 years later.[13] Other studies have observed that the expected negative relationship between M100 latency and age is either absent in ASD[15] or observed only in the left hemisphere.[33] Finally, in comparison with TD controls, individuals with ASD demonstrate a reduced right hemisphere dynamic range (∼6 ms) indicating reduced sensitivity to spectral contrasts.[9]

Of clinical interest is the relationship between neurophysiology and behavior. Because efficient processing of auditory input is crucial for developing language, measuring neurophysiological responses to sound in individuals with ASD offers insight into how differences in brain function affect behavior. There is some evidence that M50 predicts language impairment.[34] This, however, has not been found across studies.[15] A delayed M100 latency has also been associated with language impairment in ASD; however, it is not reflective of idiopathic language impairment.[35] Recent data from Roberts and colleagues[36] suggested that profoundly delayed M50 and M100 latencies are found in individuals with ASD who are minimally verbal/nonverbal compared with TD children and higher functioning children with ASD (Fig. 1). Nonetheless, the specificity of M50/M100 delays for language versus cognitive impairments has not been clearly established.

Magnetic Mismatch Field

The auditory electroencephalogram recorded mismatch negativity (MMN) and its MEG equivalent, the magnetic mismatch field (MMF), are neurophysiological indices of auditory change detection.[37–39] During a train of standard sounds, the MMN/F occurs in response to an unexpected deviant stimulus (eg, /ɑ/, /ɑ/, /ɑ/, /u/) that violates sensory expectation.[38,40] Therefore, the MMN/F has been proposed as an index of auditory memory.[38,41] In adults, the MMN occurs between 170 and 250 ms poststimulus onset, even in the absence of overt attention to the stimulus.[38] MMN can be elicited by a change in pitch, duration, or intensity,[38,40] and can even occur as a function of interstimulus interval (ISI) change.[42] In experiments involving newborns, auditory MMN latency is slightly later[43–46] and MMN amplitude smaller[44,47] than in older children and adults. MMN latency corresponds to an adult-like latency by the time children are school age.[48,49] Research has shown that auditory MMF signals originate from the temporoparietal cortex and dorsolateral

prefrontal cortex.[41,50] The difference wave, which permits the most robust identification of the MMN component, is identified by subtracting mean responses to deviant stimuli from mean responses to standard stimuli.[51]

MEG studies using the MMF have explored auditory perception of tones and speech sounds in children on the autism spectrum. School-age ASD populations and adults with ASD show MMF differences in response to pure tone and vowel changes versus age-matched controls.[5,10–12,14,17,52]

Oram Cardy and colleagues[12] examined the MMF in 7 children with ASD and 9 TD children aged 8 to 17 years. During the experiment, children were presented with pure tones (300 ms; 300 and 700 Hz; ISI 400 ms) and synthesized vowels /ɑ/ and /u/ (300 ms, F_1 = 310 and 710 Hz, respectively; ISI 400 ms) in an oddball paradigm in which trains of standard stimuli were followed by intermittent deviant stimuli (standard, 85%; deviant, 15%). MMF amplitudes were not significantly different between groups; however, a delayed MMF response was found in the ASD group in response to all stimuli. The authors speculated that slower auditory change detection may be associated with language impairment in children with ASD.[12]

A study by Roberts and colleagues[14] looked at MMF responses to pure tones and vowels in 18 children with ASD and language impairment, 33

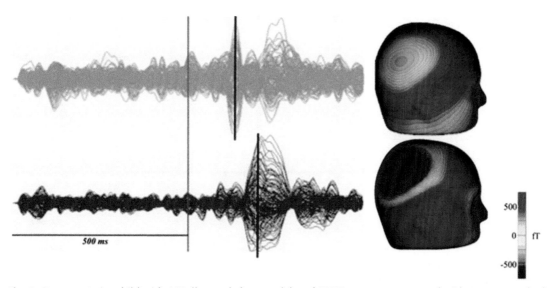

Fig. 1. Representative child with ASD (*bottom*) shows a delayed M100 response compared with an age-matched typically developing control (*top*). At left, sensor overlay plots show the auditory evoked response from a typically developing child (*green*) and a child with ASD (*purple*). The stimulus onset is marked in gray and the M100 response shown with the black line. At right, M100 magnetic field maps (*top*, TD; *bottom*, ASD). (*From* RG Port, AR Anwar, M Ku, et al. Prospective MEG biomarkers in ASD: pre-clinical evidence and clinical promise of electrophysiological signatures. Yale J Biol Med 2015. Mar 4;88(1): p.27; with permission.)

children with ASD without language impairment, and 27 age-matched comparison children (8–11 years). Tone and vowel stimuli were the same as those reported by Oram Cardy and colleagues.[12] In both the tone and vowel condition, the authors found a significantly later MMF latency in the full sample of children with ASD compared with TD peers, and a significantly later MMF latency in children with ASD and concomitant language impairment compared with children with ASD without language impairment. These findings coincide with those of Oram Cardy and colleagues[12] and offer further evidence that auditory perceptual differences in ASD and language impairment are not specific to speech sounds but also apply to simple tones. Using receiver operator characteristic analysis, the authors tested the sensitivity and specificity of mean MMF latency as a diagnostic indicator of language impairment in ASD. Sensitivity was found to be 82.4% and specificity was 71.2%.[14] These results were again replicated with an additional cohort of 8- to 12-year-old minimally verbal/nonverbal children with ASD,[11] as well as in young adults with ASD during an auditory oddball paradigm with vowel stimuli.[10]

Although delayed MMF latency has been associated with language impairment across studies, further research is needed to determine if MMF is associated primarily with language impairment concomitant with ASD or with general language impairment/delay (**Fig. 2**). A small study by Roberts and colleagues[35] suggested that similar MMF delays were observed in specific language impairment, suggesting that MMF latency delay is associated with language impairment, independent of ASD diagnosis. A recent study showing MMF latency delay in boys with 47,XYY syndrome (independent of ASD diagnosis) also supported the general association of MMF latency delay with language impairment.[53]

Auditory Gamma-Band Activity

Auditory gamma-band STG activity has also been proposed as a marker of ASD. In TD individuals gamma-band steady-state responses can be observed following trains of auditory stimuli (tones, clicks) and reflect local connectivity. Steady-state gamma is greatest when auditory stimuli are modulated at 40 Hz,[54–57] with the primary steady-state auditory generators in left and right primary/

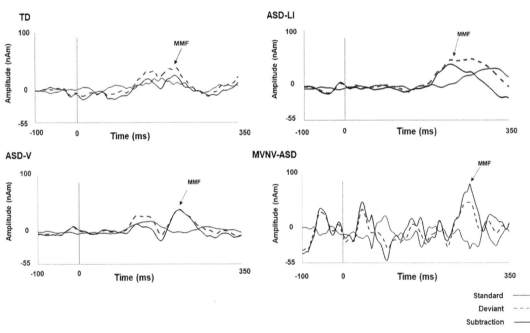

Fig. 2. Source response waveforms from superior temporal gyrus. Vertical lines indicate stimulus onset (0 ms). Arrows indicate MMF latency in a representative TD child (182 ms), verbal ASD without language impairment (214 ms), ASD and language impairment (222 ms), and ASD minimally verbal/nonverbal (MVNV) (270 ms). The solid gray line indicates the standard response, the dashed gray line indicates the deviant response, and the solid black line their subtraction to yield the difference wave. (*From* Matsuzaki, J., E. S. Kuschner, L. Blaskey, et al. Abnormal auditory mismatch fields are associated with communication impairment in both verbal and minimally verbal/nonverbal children who have autism spectrum disorder. Autism Res 2019. Aug;12(8):1225-1235; with permission.)

secondary auditory cortex.[58] Differences in post-stimulus auditory gamma-band activity have been found in individuals with ASD compared with those with typical development[7,13,58–61] as well as in first-degree relatives of individuals with ASD.[62,63] Wilson and colleagues[58] found reduced 40 Hz left hemisphere gamma-band activity in individuals with ASD during a 40-Hz click train task. When presenting participants with 1000-Hz tones, Rojas and colleagues[63] also found decreased bilateral 40 Hz early STG gamma-band inter-trial coherence (ITC) in adults with ASD and their parents.

In a study of 105 children with ASD and 36 TD controls, Edgar and colleagues[7] found smaller increases in bilateral gamma evoked activity from 50 to 150 ms in ASD compared with TD children in response to randomly presented sinusoidal tones (300 ms; 200, 300, 500, and 1000 Hz, ISI 1000 ms) as well as bilateral decreases in gamma ITC from 50 to 200 ms (300, 500, and 1000 Hz). Low-frequency ITC (below 20 Hz) was also decreased after 50 ms (200, 300, and 500 Hz) in ASD. With the exception of right high gamma, bilateral 30 to 50 Hz prestimulus power was greater in individuals with ASD for all stimuli. These increases in left and right 4 to 80 Hz prestimulus activity were associated with delayed M100 latency. Increased right hemisphere 30 to 50 Hz prestimulus activity as well as left hemisphere 100 Hz poststimulus gamma were associated with decreased language scores[7] (Fig. 3).

Support for the hypothesis that gamma-band oscillatory activity reflects local neural circuitry is provided by the emerging association between gamma-band activity and MRS-determined estimates of gamma-amino butyric acid (GABA), as an index of inhibitory tone.[64–68] This is particularly relevant to ASD, as the seminal work of Rubenstein and Merzenich[69] hypothesized that ASD symptomatology, at least in part, stems from an imbalance of cortical excitatory and inhibitory neurotransmission.[70] This is supported yet further by evidence of diminished GABA in ASD, with regional dependence most pronounced in temporal and posterior frontal/parietal regions.[59]

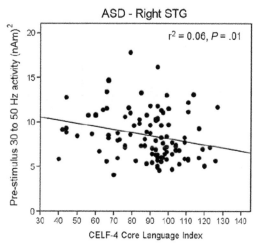

Fig. 3. Scatterplot of Clinical Evaluation of Language-Fourth Edition (CELF-4), Core language index scores (x axis) and right STG prestimulus gamma activity (y axis, 30–50 Hz) in individuals with ASD. In ASD lower CELF-4 scores were associated with increased right hemisphere prestimulus gamma activity. (*From* Edgar, J. C., S. Y. Khan, L. Blaskey, et al. Neuromagnetic oscillations predict evoked-response latency delays and core language deficits in autism spectrum disorders. J Autism Dev Disord 2015; 45(2):395-405; with permission.)

when the target word is related to the prime.[72] It has been suggested that alpha ERD is associated with lexical retrieval with larger ERDs indicating longer lexical search time.[72,75]

In a study of 51 children with ASD and 19 TD children aged 6 to 11 years, Bloy and colleagues[76] found that increased theta, alpha, and beta band (5–20 Hz) ERD 200 to 1000 ms poststimulus (word and plausible nonword) were correlated with better language assessment scores but not with ASD group allocation, symptom severity, or IQ. These results were true for words and plausible nonwords. Because a plausible nonword (eg, blick) would likely trigger a search of the lexicon similar to that of a real word, results support the use of ERD as a measure of lexical search time. Thus, 5 to 20 Hz ERDs have the potential to be used as a clinical measure of lexical access in ASD.

Auditory Alpha and Beta-Band Activity

Another promising area of research examines event-related desynchrony (ERD), or decreased synchrony within a specific frequency band following the presentation of a stimulus.[71] Studies have shown that theta, alpha, and beta ERD changes occur in response to auditory, written language, and memory tasks (Fig. 4).[72–75] Specifically during semantic priming tasks, alpha and beta ERDs are reduced 200+ ms after stimulus onset

Resting-State Alpha

Eyes-closed resting-state tasks have been used to study neural oscillations in ASD. Oscillatory activity results from large numbers of simultaneously firing neurons, and is thought to mediate a broad spectrum of cortical activity (for reviews see Uhlhaas and colleagues[77] and Wang[78]). Alpha oscillations (8–13 Hz) are the dominant brain oscillation during the eyes-closed resting state.[7,79–81] Resting-state alpha activity is most prominent in

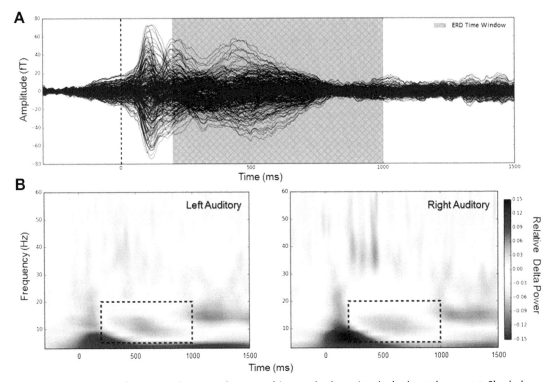

Fig. 4. (*A*) Sensory waveforms grand averaged across subject and token, time locked to token onset. Shaded area (*red*) indicates the time window used in ERD measurements. (*B*) Grand average spectro-temporal plots (time-frequency representations) for the left and right auditory cortex source locations. (*From* L Bloy, K Shwayder, L Blaskey, et al. A Spectrotemporal Correlate of Language Impairment in Autism Spectrum Disorder. J Autism Dev Disord 2019; Aug 49(8): 3181-3190; with permission.)

parietal-occipital regions,[81–84] and alpha activity increases as a function of age in TD individuals.[85–96] MEG studies have isolated parietal-occipital regions, especially near primary visual cortex, as the area with the strongest resting-state alpha generators.[81,84,97,98] Several studies have shown differences in resting-state alpha activity in children with ASD compared with TD individuals.[7,99,100]

Cornew and colleagues[99] explored resting-state activity in 27 children with ASD and 23 TD children aged 6 to 15 years. Findings included increased delta, theta, and high frequency power in ASD. Alpha power, specifically in the temporal and parietal regions, was also increased in ASD compared with TD, and these increases were correlated with ASD symptoms.[99] Edgar and colleagues[7] assessed alpha activity in 41 children with ASD and 47 TD children aged 6 to 14 years. Results demonstrated increased alpha activity bordering the central sulcus and parietal association cortices in ASD versus TD.

Increased alpha activity is also of clinical interest, with increased deficits in social

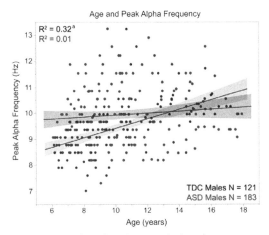

Fig. 5. Scatterplots showing associations between age (x axis) and peak alpha frequency (y axis) for 121 typically developing children (TDC) (*blue*) and 183 children with ASD (*red*). A significant interaction term indicated group slope differences. [a] *P*<.001. (*From* JC Edgar, M Dipiero, E McBride, et al. Abnormal maturation of the resting-state peak alpha frequency in children with autism spectrum disorder. Hum Brain Mapp 2019. Aug 1;40(11):3288-3298; with permission.)

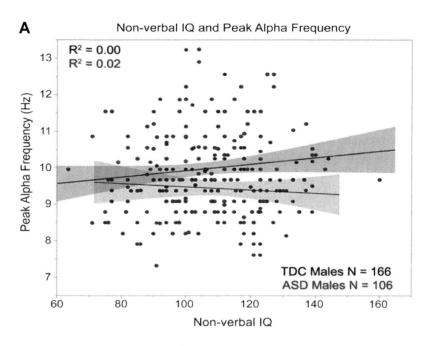

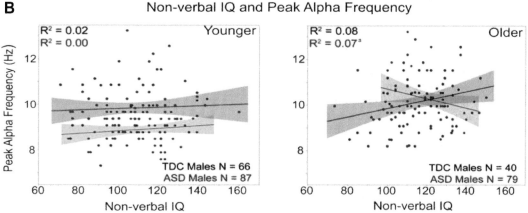

Fig. 6. (A) Scatterplots showing associations between nonverbal IQ (x axis) and peak alpha frequency (y axis) for TDC (blue) and ASD (red). (B) Nonverbal IQ and peak alpha frequency associations shown for the younger (<10 years old; left plot) and older children (>10 years old; right plot). [a] $P<.05$. (From JC Edgar, M Dipiero, E McBride, et al. Abnormal maturation of the resting-state peak alpha frequency in children with autism spectrum disorder. Hum Brain Mapp 2019. Aug 1;40(11):3288-3298; with permission.)

responsiveness associated with increased left central sulcus alpha activity and with more typical social behaviors associated with greater calcarine region alpha activity in ASD. Also of interest, peak alpha frequency did not increase with age in individuals with ASD, indicating abnormal patterns of alpha maturation in ASD compared with TD children.[7] These peak alpha frequency results were replicated in a large cohort of male children (ASD, 183; TD, 121) aged 6 to 17 years, with peak alpha frequency group differences most prominent in the younger children with ASD than the TD children (6–10 years) (Fig. 5). Additionally,

the same study found a positive association between peak alpha frequency and verbal IQ in older individuals with ASD, while the reverse pattern was observed in older TD children (Fig. 6).[100]

POTENTIAL FUTURE ROLES FOR MAGNETOENCEPHALOGRAPHY IN THE CLINICAL MANAGEMENT OF AUTISM SPECTRUM DISORDER

Until recently, MEG research has focused on older children and adults. However, the recent development of MEG scanners with a sensor helmet sized for young infants is resulting in a greater number of MEG infant studies. Longitudinal research on infants at risk for ASD (baby siblings of children with ASD) is needed to determine if the neurophysiological differences found in school-age children with ASD are apparent before a child is formally diagnosed with ASD. If infant MEG measures are found to predict language and ASD outcomes at age 3 years, these measures could be developed into diagnostic or predictive measures for infants.

It is of note that, to date, MEG ASD studies have focused on reporting group differences. Although these studies are necessary to show research directions worth pursuing, MEG markers will need to show good sensitivity and specificity to be of clinical use. To this end, the use of normative databases (with concomitant standardization of data collection and analysis methods) is needed to determine if individuals with ASD can be identified at the individual level. It is also likely that multiple MEG measures (auditory, visual, social, resting state) can be combined to predict ASD with more accuracy than a single measure, with machine learning approaches used to identify the combination of measures that best differentiate infants and children with and without ASD.

MEG markers may also offer prognostic information (eg, will a child have difficulty developing language?) and thus allow targeted treatment (behavioral and pharmaceutical), based on an individual's neurophysiological profile. MEG also has the potential to assess the efficacy of ASD treatments; via determining if brain neural activity is changing in response to treatment, clinicians may be better positioned to decide whether to continue or terminate treatment.

To conclude, although more research is needed before clinical MEG examinations are available for ASD, current MEG research suggests several markers of clinical interest. Work is needed to identify diagnostic or prognostic ASD markers that provide good sensitivity and specificity at the individual level.

REFERENCES

1. Kanner L. Autistic disturbances of affective contact. Nervous Child 1943;2:217–50.
2. American Psychiatric Association. Diagnostic and statistical manual of mental disorders: DSM-5. 5th edition. Arlington (VA): American Psychiatric Publishing, Inc; 2013.
3. Kogan MD, Vladutiu CJ, Schieve LA, et al. The prevalence of parent-reported autism spectrum disorder among US children. Pediatrics 2018;142 [pii:e20174161].
4. Baio J, Wiggins L, Chistenson DL, et al. Prevalence of autism spectrum disorder among children aged 8 years—autism and developmental disabilities monitoring network, 11 sites, United States,2014. MMWR Surveill Summ 2018;67:1–23.
5. Berman JI, Edgar JC, Blaskey L, et al. Multimodal diffusion-MRI and MEG assessment of auditory and language system development in autism spectrum disorder. Front Neuroanat 2016;10:30.
6. Edgar JC, Fisk Iv CL, Berman JI, et al. Auditory encoding abnormalities in children with autism spectrum disorder suggest delayed development of auditory cortex. Mol Autism 2015a;6:69.
7. Edgar JC, Khan SY, Blaskey L, et al. Neuromagnetic oscillations predict evoked-response latency delays and core language deficits in autism spectrum disorders. J Autism Dev Disord 2015b;45: 395–405.
8. Edgar JC, Lanza MR, Daina AB, et al. Missing and delayed auditory responses in young and older children with autism spectrum disorders. Front Hum Neurosci 2014;8:417.
9. Gage NM, Siegel B, Callen M, et al. Cortical sound processing in children with autism disorder: an MEG investigation. Neuroreport 2003a;14:2047–51.
10. Matsuzaki J, Ku M, Berman JI, et al. Abnormal auditory mismatch fields in adults with autism spectrum disorder. Neurosci Lett 2019a;698:140–5.
11. Matsuzaki J, Kuschner ES, Blaskey L, et al. Abnormal auditory mismatch fields are associated with communication impairment in both verbal and minimally verbal/nonverbal children who have autism spectrum disorder. Autism Res 2019b; 12(8):1225–35.
12. Oram Cardy JE, Flagg EJ, Roberts W, et al. Delayed mismatch field for speech and nonspeech sounds in children with autism. Neuroreport 2005b;16:521–5.
13. Port RG, Anwar AR, Ku M, et al. Prospective MEG biomarkers in ASD: pre-clinical evidence and clinical promise of electrophysiological signatures. Yale J Biol Med 2015;88:25–36.
14. Roberts TP, Cannon KM, Tavabi K, et al. Auditory magnetic mismatch field latency: a biomarker for language impairment in autism. Biol Psychiatry 2011;70:263–9.
15. Roberts TP, Khan SY, Rey M, et al. MEG detection of delayed auditory evoked responses in autism spectrum disorders: towards an imaging biomarker for autism. Autism Res 2010;3:8–18.
16. Roberts TP, Lanza MR, Dell J, et al. Maturational differences in thalamocortical white matter microstructure and auditory evoked response latencies in autism spectrum disorders. Brain Res 2013; 1537:79–85.
17. Yoshimura Y, Kikuchi M, Hayashi N, et al. Altered human voice processing in the frontal cortex and

a developmental language delay in 3- to 5-year-old children with autism spectrum disorder. Sci Rep 2017;7:17116.

18. Hari R. The neuromagnetic method in the study of the human auditory cortex. In: Grandori F, Hoke M, Romani GL, editors. Auditory evoked magnetic fields and potentials advances in audiology. Basel (Switzerland): Karger; 1990. p. 222–82.

19. Lütkenhöner B, Steinsträter O. High-precision neuromagnetic study of the functional organization of the human auditory cortex. Audiol Neurootol 1998;3:191–213.

20. Oram Cardy JE, Flagg EJ, Roberts W, et al. Magnetoencephalography identifies rapid temporal processing deficit in autism and language impairment. Neuroreport 2005;16:329–32.

21. Paetau R, Ahonen A, Salonen O, et al. Auditory evoked magnetic fields to tones and pseudowords in healthy children and adults. J Clin Neurophysiol 1995;12:177–85.

22. Ponton CW, Eggermont JJ, Kwong B, et al. Maturation of human central auditory system activity: evidence from multi-channel evoked potentials. Clin Neurophysiol 2000;111:220–36.

23. Roberts TP, Ferrari P, Stufflebeam SM, et al. Latency of the auditory evoked neuromagnetic field components: stimulus dependence and insights toward perception. J Clin Neurophysiol 2000;17:114–29.

24. Roberts TP, Poeppel D. Latency of auditory evoked M100 as a function of tone frequency. Neuroreport 1996;7:1138–40.

25. Wunderlich JL, Cone-Wesson BK. Maturation of CAEP in infants and children: a review. Hear Res 2006;212:212–23.

26. Huotilainen M, Winkler I, Alho K, et al. Combined mapping of human auditory EEG and MEG responses. Electroencephalogr Clin Neurophysiol 1998;108:370–9.

27. Mäkelä JP, Hämäläinen M, Hari R, et al. Wholehead mapping of middle-latency auditory evoked magnetic fields. Electroencephalogr Clin Neurophysiol 1994;92:414–21.

28. Pelizzone M, Hari R, Mäkelä JP, et al. Cortical origin of middle-latency auditory evoked responses in man. Neurosci Lett 1987;82:303–7.

29. Reite M, Teale P, Zimmerman J, et al. Source location of a 50 msec latency auditory evoked field component. Electroencephalogr Clin Neurophysiol 1988;70:490–8.

30. Yoshiura T, Ueno S, Iramina K, et al. Source localization of middle latency auditory evoked magnetic fields. Brain Res 1995;703:139–44.

31. Yvert B, Crouzeix A, Bertrand O, et al. Multiple supratemporal sources of magnetic and electric auditory evoked middle latency components in humans. Cereb Cortex 2001;11:411–23.

32. Matsuzaki J, Kagitani-Shimono K, Goto T, et al. Differential responses of primary auditory cortex in autistic spectrum disorder with auditory hypersensitivity. Neuroreport 2012;23:113–8.

33. Gage NM, Siegel B, Roberts TP. Cortical auditory system maturational abnormalities in children with autism disorder: an MEG investigation. Brain Res Dev Brain Res 2003b;144:201–9.

34. Oram Cardy JE, Flagg EJ, Roberts W, et al. Auditory evoked fields predict language ability and impairment in children. Int J Psychophysiol 2008;68:170–5.

35. Roberts TP, Heiken K, Kahn SY, et al. Delayed magnetic mismatch negativity field, but not auditory M100 response, in specific language impairment. Neuroreport 2012;23:463–8.

36. Roberts TP, Matsuzaki J, Blaskey L, et al. 2019. Delayed M50/M100 latency arising from superior temporal gyrus in minimally verbal/nonverbal children. In International Society for Autism Research. Montreal, Canada, May 4, 2019.

37. Näätänen R, Gaillard AW, Mäntysalo S. Early selective-attention effect on evoked potential reinterpreted. Acta Psychol (Amst) 1978;42:313–29.

38. Näätänen R, Paavilainen P, Rinne T, et al. The mismatch negativity (MMN) in basic research of central auditory processing: a review. Clin Neurophysiol 2007;118:2544–90.

39. Schwartz S, Shinn-Cunningham B, Tager-Flusberg H. Meta-analysis and systematic review of the literature characterizing auditory mismatch negativity in individuals with autism. Neurosci Biobehav Rev 2018;87:106–17.

40. Näätänen R. Attention and brain function. Hillsdale (NJ): Erlbaum; 1992.

41. Alho K. Cerebral generators of mismatch negativity (MMN) and its magnetic counterpart (MMNm) elicited by sound changes. Ear Hear 1995;16:38–51.

42. Ford JM, Hillyard SA. Event-related potentials (ERPs) to interruptions of a steady rhythm. Psychophysiology 1981;18:322–30.

43. Cheour M, Ceponiene R, Lehtokoski A, et al. Development of language-specific phoneme representations in the infant brain. Nat Neurosci 1998;1:351–3.

44. Cheour M, Alho K, Saino K, et al. The mismatch negativity to changes in speech sounds at the age of three months. Dev Neuropsychol 1997;13:167–74.

45. Cheour-Luhtanen M, Alho K, Sainio K, et al. The ontogenetically earliest discriminative response of the human brain. Psychophysiology 1996;33:478–81.

46. Kurtzberg D, Vaughan HG Jr, Kreuzer JA, et al. Developmental studies and clinical applications of mismatch negativity: Problems and prospects. Ear Hear 1995;16:105–17.

47. Aaltonen O, Niemi P, Nyrke T, et al. Event-related brain potentials and the perception of a phonetic continuum. Biol Psychol 1987;24:197–207.

48. Csépe V. On the origin and development of the mismatch negativity. Ear Hear 1995;16:91–104.

49. Kraus N, McGee T, Sharma A, et al. Mismatch negativity event-related potential elicited by speech stimuli. Ear Hear 1992;13:158–64.

50. Handy TE. Event-related potentials: a methods handbook. Cambridge (MA): MIT Press; 2005.

51. Luck SJ. An introduction to event-related potential technique. Cambridge (MA): MIT Press; 2005.

52. Matsuzaki J, Kagitani-Shimono K, Sugata H, et al. Delayed mismatch field latencies in autism spectrum disorder with abnormal auditory sensitivity: a magnetoencephalographic study. Front Hum Neurosci 2017;11:446.

53. Matsuzaki J, Bloy L, Blaskey L, et al. Abnormal Auditory Mismatch Fields in Children and Adolescents with 47, XYY Syndrome. Dev Neurosci 2019;41(1–2):123–31.

54. Boettcher FA, Madhotra D, Poth EA, et al. The frequency-modulation following response in young and aged human subjects. Hear Res 2002;165:10–8.

55. Boettcher FA, Poth EA, Mills JH, et al. The amplitude-modulation following response in young and aged human subjects. Hear Res 2001;153:32–42.

56. Hari R, Hämäläinen M, Joutsiniemi SL. Neuromagnetic steady-state responses to auditory stimuli. J Acoust Soc Am 1989;86:1033–9.

57. Stapells DR, Linden D, Suffield JB, et al. Human auditory steady state potentials. Ear Hear 1984;5:105–13.

58. Wilson TW, Rojas DC, Reite ML, et al. Children and adolescents with autism exhibit reduced MEG steady-state gamma responses. Biol Psychiatry 2007;62:192–7.

59. Gaetz W, Bloy L, Wang DJ, et al. GABA estimation in the brains of children on the autism spectrum: measurement precision and regional cortical variation. Neuroimage 2014;86:1–9.

60. Gandal MJ, Edgar JC, Ehrlichman RS, et al. Validating γ oscillations and delayed auditory responses as translational biomarkers of autism. Biol Psychiatry 2010;68:1100–6.

61. Tanigawa J, Kagitani-Shimono K, Matsuzaki J, et al. Atypical auditory language processing in adolescents with autism spectrum disorder. Clin Neurophysiol 2018;129:2029–37.

62. McFadden KL, Hepburn S, Winterrowd E, et al. Abnormalities in gamma-band responses to language stimuli in first-degree relatives of children with autism spectrum disorder: an MEG study. BMC Psychiatry 2012;12:213.

63. Rojas DC, Maharajh K, Teale P, et al. Reduced neural synchronization of gamma-band MEG oscillations in first-degree relatives of children with autism. BMC Psychiatry 2008;8:66.

64. Balz J, Keil J, Roa Romero Y, et al. GABA concentration in superior temporal sulcus predicts gamma power and perception in the sound-induced flash illusion. Neuroimage 2016;125:724–30.

65. Edden RA, Muthukumaraswamy SD, Freeman TC, et al. Orientation discrimination performance is predicted by GABA concentration and gamma oscillation frequency in human primary visual cortex. J Neurosci 2009;29:15721–6.

66. Gaetz W, Edgar JC, Wang DJ, et al. Relating MEG measured motor cortical oscillations to resting γ-aminobutyric acid (GABA) concentration. Neuroimage 2011;55:616–21.

67. Muthukumaraswamy SD, Edden RA, Jones DK, et al. Resting GABA concentration predicts peak gamma frequency and fMRI amplitude in response to visual stimulation in humans. Proc Natl Acad Sci U S A 2009;106:8356–61.

68. Port RG, Gaetz W, Bloy L, et al. Exploring the relationship between cortical GABA concentrations, auditory gamma-band responses and development in ASD: evidence for an altered maturational trajectory in ASD. Autism Res 2017;10:593–607.

69. Rubenstein JL, Merzenich MM. Model of autism: increased ratio of excitation/inhibition in key neural systems. Genes Brain Behav 2003;2:255–67.

70. Port RG, Oberman LM, Roberts TP. Revisiting the excitation/inhibition imbalance hypothesis of ASD through a clinical lens. Br J Radiol 2019;92:20180944.

71. Neuper C, Pfurtscheller G. Event-related dynamics of cortical rhythms: frequency-specific features and functional correlates. Int J Psychophysiol 2001;43:41–58.

72. Brennan J, Lignos C, Embick D, et al. Spectro-temporal correlates of lexical access during auditory lexical decision. Brain Lang 2014;133:39–46.

73. Krause CM, Pesonen M, Hämäläinen H. Brain oscillatory responses during the different stages of an auditory memory search task in children. Neuroreport 2007;18:213–6.

74. Pesonen M, Björnberg CH, Hämäläinen H, et al. Brain oscillatory 1–30 Hz EEG ERD/ERS responses during the different stages of an auditory memory search task. Neurosci Lett 2006;399:45–50.

75. Tavabi K, Embick D, Roberts TP. Spectral-temporal analysis of cortical oscillations during lexical processing. Neuroreport 2011;22:474–8.

76. Bloy L, Shwayder K, Blaskey L, et al. A spectrotemporal correlate of language impairment in autism spectrum disorder. J Autism Dev Disord 2019;49:3181–90.

77. Uhlhaas PJ, Pipa G, Lima B, et al. Neural synchrony in cortical networks: history, concept and current status. Front Integr Neurosci 2009;3:17.

78. Wang XJ. Neurophysiological and computational principles of cortical rhythms in cognition. Physiol Rev 2010;90:1195–268.

79. Berger H. Hans Berger on the electroencephalogram of man. Archiv für Psychiatrie und Nervenkrankheiten 1929;87:527–70.

80. Haegens S, Cousijn H, Wallis G, et al. Inter- and intra-individual variability in alpha peak frequency. Neuroimage 2014;92:46–55.

81. Hari R, Salmelin R. Human cortical oscillations: a neuromagnetic view through the skull. Trends Neurosci 1997;20:44–9.

82. Ciulla C, Takeda T, Endo H. MEG characterization of spontaneous alpha rhythm in the human brain. Brain Topogr 1999;11:211–22.

83. Niedermeyer E. Maturation of the EEG: development of waking and sleep patterns. In: Niedermeyer E, Lopes da Silva FH, editors. Electroencephalography: basic principles, clinical applications, and related fields. Baltimore (MD): Williams and Wilkins; 1993. p. 167–91.

84. Salmelin R, Hari R. Characterization of spontaneous MEG rhythms in healthy adults. Electroencephalogr Clin Neurophysiol 1994;91:237–48.

85. Alvarez Amador A, Valdés Sosa PA, Pascual Marqui RD, et al. On the structure of EEG development. Electroencephalogr Clin Neurophysiol 1989; 73:10–9.

86. Chiang AK, Rennie CJ, Robinson PA, et al. Age trends and sex differences of alpha rhythms including split alpha peaks. Clin Neurophysiol 2011;122:1505–17.

87. Cragg L, Kovacevic N, McIntosh AR, et al. Maturation of EEG power spectra in early adolescence: a longitudinal study. Dev Sci 2011;14:935–43.

88. Epstein HT. EEG developmental stages. Dev Psychobiol 1980;13:621–31.

89. Gibbs FA, Knott JR. Growth of the electrical activity of the cortex. Electroencephalogr Clin Neurophysiol 1949;1:223–9.

90. Hughes JR. Normal limits of the EEG. In: Halliday RM, Butler SR, Paul R, editors. A textbook of clinical neurophysiology. New York: Wiley; 1987. p. 105–54.

91. John ER, Ahn H, Prichep L, et al. Developmental equations for the electroencephalogram. Science 1980;210:1255–8.

92. Klimesch W. EEG alpha and theta oscillations reflect cognitive and memory performance: a review and analysis. Brain Res Rev 1999;29:169–95.

93. Miskovic V, Ma X, Chou CA, et al. Developmental changes in spontaneous electrocortical activity and network organization from early to late childhood. Neuroimage 2015;118:237–47.

94. Niedermeyer E. The normal EEG of the waking adult. In: Niedermeyer E, Lopes da Silva FH, editors. Electroencephalography: basic principles, clinical applications, and related fields. Baltimore (MD): Williams and Wilkins; 1993. p. 167–91.

95. Somsen RJ, van't Klooster BJ, van der Molen MW, et al. Growth spurts in brain maturation during middle childhood as indexed by EEG power spectra. Biol Psychol 1997;44:187–209.

96. Stroganova TA, Orekhova EV, Posikera IN. EEG alpha rhythm in infants. Clin Neurophysiol 1999; 110:997–1012.

97. Bouyer JJ, Tilquin C, Rougeul A. Thalamic rhythms in cat during quiet wakefulness and immobility. Electroencephalogr Clin Neurophysiol 1983;55: 180–7.

98. Huang MX, Huang CW, Robb A, et al. MEG source imaging method using fast L1 minimum-norm and its applications to signals with brain noise and human resting-state source amplitude images. Neuroimage 2014;84:585–604.

99. Cornew L, Roberts TP, Blaskey L, et al. Resting-state oscillatory activity in autism spectrum disorders. J Autism Dev Disord 2012;42:1884–94.

100. Edgar JC, Dipiero M, McBride E, et al. Abnormal maturation of the resting-state peak alpha frequency in children with autism spectrum disorder. Hum Brain Mapp 2019;40(11):3288–98.

Magnetoencephalography for Schizophrenia

J. Christopher Edgar, PhD[a],*, Anika Guha, MA[b], Gregory A. Miller, PhD[b,c]

KEYWORDS

• Schizophrenia • Neuroimaging • Magnetoencephalography • Neuroradiologists

KEY POINTS

- This article on schizophrenia considers the possible future clinical use of magnetoencephalography (MEG) by radiologists via focusing on areas of active research: research studies examining whole-brain resting-state activity, studies examining auditory encoding processes, and studies examining functional connectivity.
- Rather than provide a comprehensive review, this article considers the types of MEG images that neuroradiologists might one day read as part of a clinical radiology schizophrenia examination.
- The use of normative whole-brain MEG databases to identify abnormality at the individual level is highlighted, a procedure that allows for a more quantitative assessment of neural activity.
- The clinical payoff in examining activity throughout the brain is identifying abnormalities specific to each patient (eg, observing abnormalities in superior temporal gyrus or frontal lobes), with individual findings hopefully one day guiding diagnosis and treatment.

Although radiologists have a large arsenal of imaging tools at their disposal (including x-ray, computed tomography, MR imaging, and ultrasound), these tools are not routinely used for clinical assessment of schizophrenia (Sz).[1–6] Indeed, although increased ventricular volume[7–9] and reduced superior temporal gyrus gray matter[10–12] in Sz are robust findings at the group level, brain imaging does not provide clinically useable information (diagnostic or prognostic) regarding Sz at the individual level due to insufficient sensitivity and specificity. As such, the relatively uncommon radiology clinical referral of someone having or suspected of having Sz is to rule out conditions such as a brain tumor or encephalitis.

Magnetoencephalography (MEG) has been used for more than 25 years in research studies examining neural activity in Sz. Although abnormalities in resting-state activity as well as basic sensory processing and cognitive processes are reliably reported in MEG studies,[13–22] analogous to other brain imaging modalities, no MEG marker for Sz exists for use at the individual level. MEG provides the ability to investigate brain activity at specific brain regions as well as to create whole-brain 3-dimensional (3D) images from the MEG sensor data. As radiologists excel at interpreting 3D brain images, neuroradiologists are well placed to make good use of MEG brain images. However, as detailed throughout this article, the MEG brain images of interest for Sz will be different from the structural brain images neuroradiologists typically encounter. This is because MEG records brain neural activity, and thus MEG brain images are images of brain function rather than brain structure. Although functional MR (fMR) imaging clinical studies are sometimes obtained by radiologists, MEG images differ from fMR images, as MEG

Funded by: NIHHYB. Grant number(s): R01 MH107506; R01 MH110544S1; R21 MH098204; R21 NS090192.
[a] Department of Radiology, Research Division, Children's Hospital of Philadelphia, 3401 Civic Center Boulevard, 1st Floor, Room 115A, Philadelphia, PA 19104, USA; [b] Department of Psychology, University of California, Los Angeles, Franz Hall, 502 Portola Plaza, Los Angeles, CA 90095, USA; [c] Department of Psychiatry and Biobehavioral Sciences, University of California, Los Angeles, Los Angeles, CA 90095, USA
* Corresponding author.
E-mail address: edgarj@email.chop.edu

records neural activity directly, in "real time," rather than time-delayed and time-blurred hemodynamic activity related to neural activity, and thus millisecond-by-millisecond images (or even movies) are potentially available with MEG.

This article on Sz considers the possible future use of MEG by radiologists via focusing on areas of active research: research studies examining whole-brain resting-state activity, studies examining auditory encoding processes, and studies examining functional connectivity. Rather than provide a comprehensive review, this article considers the types of MEG images that neuroradiologists might one day read as part of a clinical radiology Sz examination. Given significant heterogeneity in Sz due to individual differences in genetic risk,[23,24] environmental risk,[25,26] and symptoms,[27] the brain neural abnormalities observed across individuals with Sz are likely to differ considerably. Indeed, growing clinical research evidence indicates that traditionally diagnosed Sz is diverse in cause and heterogeneous in clinical presentation. Attention is turning to specific symptoms and risk factors as potential clinical targets for detection, diagnosis, and preventive and ameliorative intervention.[28-31] The clinical payoff in examining activity throughout the brain is identifying abnormalities specific to each patient (eg, observing abnormalities in superior temporal gyrus or frontal lobes), with individual findings hopefully one day guiding diagnosis and treatment. In addition, given that it is unlikely that brain pathology in Sz will be easily observed, the use of normative whole-brain MEG databases to identify abnormality at the individual level is highlighted, a procedure that allows for a more quantitative assessment of neural activity.

RESTING-STATE ACTIVITY IN SCHIZOPHRENIA

Information related to collecting MEG data and obtaining source images is provided in Matti Hämäläinen and colleagues' article, "MEG Signal Processing, Forward Modeling, MEG Inverse Source Imaging, and Coherence Analysis"; and Susan M. Bowyer and colleagues' article, "Pre-surgical Functional Mapping with Magnetoencephalography (MEG)"; and Mingxiong Huang and colleagues' article, "Magnetoencephalography for Mild TBI and PTSD", in this issue discuss resting-state recordings. Briefly, research studies examining resting-state (RS) brain activity in SZ typically collect spontaneous MEG in continuous 5-minute segments in an awake state. Given greater artifact in patients with Sz than in controls, multiple RS recordings are typically obtained in order to have a sufficient amount of artifact-free RS data.[32]

Although MEG Sz research has focused on RS brain activity across different frequency ranges such as alpha (9–12 Hz) and gamma (30–50 Hz),[22,33-36] RS low-frequency (delta and theta) oscillatory activity has received the most attention. Studies examining delta (1–4 Hz) and theta (4–8 Hz) activity in Sz have built on MEG and electroencephalogram (EEG) studies observing more delta and theta RS activity in Sz than controls,[33,37-43] with a meta-analysis concluding that enhanced low-frequency activity in SZ is a robust finding.[44] Given increased low-frequency activity during the waking state in Sz and given that individuals with Sz typically do not show frank pathology on structural MR images, it has been suggested that portions of the brain in Sz tend to be in an inactive, "sleep-like state"[45,46] or that slowing in Sz reflects subtle brain pathology manifested in low-frequency MEG.

Rather than merely examining low-frequency activity at the sensor level (EEG or MEG), the brain areas associated with such slowing can be identified via source localization (typically coregistering MEG data with anatomic MR imaging data). Several MEG studies have examined RS low-frequency activity throughout the brain in Sz, using one of many source-localization methods that can be used to obtain a map of RS theta activity. Using L2-minimum norm estimate localization, Fehr and colleagues[37] observed higher frontotemporal and posterior delta/theta activity in Sz than in adult controls. Using frequency-domain vector-based spatio-temporal analysis using L1-minimum norm (VESTAL[47,48]), as shown in **Fig. 1**, Chen and colleagues[49] observed abnormal low-frequency theta activity in frontal and temporo-parietal regions in adults with Sz.

A few general features of the whole-brain RS theta images in **Fig. 1** are of note. To obtain an RS theta 3D map for each subject, each subject's RS eyes-closed data were filtered to examine theta activity (4–8 Hz). To this end, the MEG continuous raw data were divided into 2.5-s epochs, which provided 0.40 Hz resolution. Epochs were overlapped 50% to adjust for windowing of each epoch. For each epoch, a fast fourier transform provided a measure of theta activity (summed across 4 Hz–8 Hz). The frequency-domain VESTAL source grid (5 mm isotropic resolution) was obtained by sampling gray-matter areas from the T1-weighted MR imaging of each subject. The sensor-space frequency-domain data were used by frequency-domain VESTAL to obtain the theta amplitude (root mean squared) at each source location. These values were then used to generate MEG theta source images for each subject. Additional details of

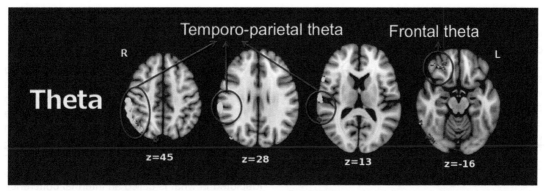

Fig. 1. Between-group VEctor-based Spatio-Temporal analysis using L1-minimum norm (VESTAL) analyses for theta (4 Hz to 8 Hz). Clusters in yellow/red show more right-hemisphere slow-wave activity in the Sz group than in the control group (*P*<.05, family-wise corrected). (*Adapted from* Chen YH, Stone-Howell B, Edgar JC, et al. Frontal slow-wave activity as a predictor of negative symptoms, cognition and functional capacity in schizophrenia. Br J Psychiatry 2016;208(2):160-7; with permission.)

frequency-domain VESTAL source imaging are provided in the article by Huang and colleagues[47] and in Mingxiong Huang and colleagues' article, "Magnetoencephalography for Mild TBI and PTSD", in this issue. **Fig. 1** is thresholded to reveal areas with significant control versus patient group differences in RS theta activity, displayed as a color overlay on the anatomic MR imaging. **Fig. 1** illustrates the value of MEG in identifying region-specific functional abnormalities, with higher spatial fidelity than scalp EEG provides.

Of note, Fehr and colleagues[37] and Chen and colleagues[49] showed control and patient low-frequency differences only at the group level. Fehr and colleagues and Chen and colleagues did not show that increased low-frequency activity was observed in each of the individuals with Sz included in their samples. Some low-frequency activity is normal and observed in most nonpatient adults (see Mingxiong Huang and colleagues' article, "Magnetoencephalography for Mild TBI and PTSD", in this issue). As such, except in extreme cases (eg, very significant slowing from cortex adjacent to a tumor[50]), identification of significantly elevated low-frequency activity at the individual level is difficult and in the authors' judgment generally not ready for routine clinical use. Thus, similar to identifying abnormal low-frequency activity in individuals with mild traumatic brain injury (Mingxiong Huang and colleagues' article, "Magnetoencephalography for Mild TBI and PTSD", in this issue), an objective method is needed to identify abnormal low-frequency activity at the individual level. Using whole-brain MEG source-space measures, Wienbruch and colleagues[42] described a method to apply a Z-score–based analysis for single subjects (a similar procedure was described in Mingxiong Huang and colleagues' article, "Magnetoencephalography for Mild TBI and PTSD", in this issue). Once a normative database is established, comparison of individual data against scores from a demographically matched control group will allow fine distinctions and comparisons unattainable by clinical observation or traditional neuroimaging alone. Via this normative approach, Rockstroh and colleagues[51] reported that the spatial topography of low-frequency activity distinguishes individuals with Sz from individuals with neurotic/affective diagnoses.

In the authors' judgment, the field is ready to begin producing data bases of this sort that will have routine clinical utility. However, before assessment of low-frequency activity in Sz can be of use in the clinic, research is needed to determine how often low-frequency abnormalities are observed at the individual level in Sz. Given changes in brain activity across the lifespan, research is also needed to determine whether different RS normative databases are needed for different age groups.[52–56] Research is also needed to determine whether analogous findings are observed across source localization methods (eg, L1 and L2 source localization methods, see Matti Hämäläinen and colleagues' article, "MEG Signal Processing, Forward Modeling, MEG Inverse Source Imaging, and Coherence Analysis", in this issue) and different MEG recording systems versus whether particular methods are superior for this purpose. Finally, research is needed to determine whether abnormal low-frequency activity identified at the individual level provides sufficient sensitivity and specificity to be used to guide treatment (eg, low-frequency abnormalities at a particular brain region indicating that patient would respond best to a specific therapy) as well as predict outcome (ie, a prognostic marker).

AUDITORY STUDIES

In addition to examining RS activity in Sz, MEG is collected in paradigms where sensory stimuli are presented (eg, auditory tones, visual images). In some instances, the subject is instructed to rest while stimuli are presented. In other instances, the subject is given a task and makes a response each time a stimulus is presented (eg, a button press). MEG data are time-locked to the presentation of each stimulus and/or button press. Because the response to a single stimulus is small relative to ongoing oscillatory activity, an averaged response to repeated stimuli is often computed. Typically, more than one hundred stimuli in each condition (eg, 130 tones, 200 pictures of faces) are presented to obtain an average evoked response providing a signal-to-noise ratio sufficient for source localization.

A very large EEG and MEG literature reports on auditory encoding abnormalities in individuals with Sz, typically using either pure tone stimuli[57–63] or steady-state auditory stimuli.[13,20] As the primary generators of early auditory encoding processes are in left and right superior temporal gyrus (STG),[15,64] MEG studies have used source localization to examine auditory encoding processes in left and right STG. Fig. 2 shows an auditory evoked response to tone stimuli in the left and right auditory cortex (activity measures obtained using single-dipole source localization). The x axis shows that auditory activity is revealed at the millisecond level, and the y axis shows that the strength of the response is measured in units of nano-amps per meter. Fig. 2 arrows show the typical adult auditory evoked responses at 50 ms and 100 ms.

When there are brain areas of a priori interest, such as left and right STG auditory areas, other measures of neural activity are often obtained via computing what are often called time-frequency measures. Fig. 3 shows auditory time-frequency plots from the right STG. The time-frequency measures for this figure were obtained via computing the continuous time course for a location within the right STG and then computing from the single trials (ie, each click or tone stimulus) the average strength of the response in terms of modulation of frequency (depicted in what is called a total power or an event-related spectral perturbation plot; Fig. 3A) and the average phase of the response (depicted in what is called an intertrial coherence or phase-locking plot; Fig. 3B), with "phase" defined in trigonometric functions.

Total power plots show the pre- to poststimulus change in neural activity in terms of frequency modulation. Intertrial coherence plots show the trial-to-trial similarity in frequency-domain neural activity. Fig. 3 illustrates some general features of time-frequency plots. First, the x axis shows activity across time in milliseconds, and the y axis shows neural activity as a function of frequency. Color codes intensity of activity at a given time and frequency. As shown in Fig. 3, around 50 to 100 ms after tone onset, increased pre- to poststimulus neural activity (total power plot) and increased similarity in the trial-to-trial response (intertrial coherence plot) are observed across a wide range of frequencies. At later times, such increases are observed only in lower frequencies (4–20 Hz). The total power plot also shows at later times a decrease in pre-to poststimulus neural activity in frequencies lower than 20 Hz, with such later decreases (event-related desynchronization) observed in most sensory systems. Depending on the research question of interest, in some cases the full time-frequency plot might be examined, and in some cases a particular time and frequency region of interest is examined (eg, theta and alpha activity from 50 to 200 ms).

Another example of MEG auditory measures are whole-brain images. Chen and colleagues[57] examined auditory encoding processes in controls and patients with Sz throughout the brain. As shown in Fig. 4, Chen and colleagues observed stronger poststimulus auditory encoding activity in controls than in patients with Sz in STG regions. Chen and colleagues also recruited unaffected relatives of the patients with Sz. As shown in Fig. 4, auditory encoding abnormalities in the patients and the unaffected relatives of the patients with SZ were shared only in left SFG, thus indicating that the identification of markers in Sz must consider specific brain regions. As noted earlier, MEG shows particular promise in providing region-specific activity with high temporal resolution.

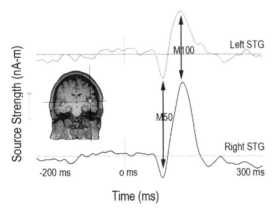

Fig. 2. Left (*green*) and right (*purple*) STG (primary/secondary auditory cortex) evoked source waveforms to tone stimuli. Arrows show typical adult auditory evoked responses at 50 ms and 100 ms.

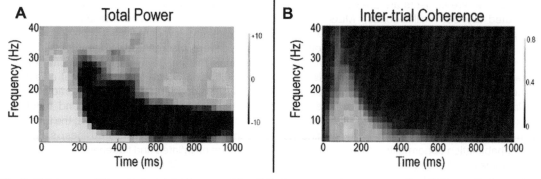

Fig. 3. Total power (*A*) and intertrial coherence (*B*) activity in response to pure tone stimuli. The x axis shows time and the y axis the percentage change in activity from baseline. The tone is presented at 0 ms.

A few aspects of the whole-brain auditory encoding image are of note. First, whereas whole-brain images of RS activity generally provide a measure of the amount of activity within a specific frequency range across the RS recordings, whole-brain evoked response images focus on a particular time period. For example, **Fig. 4** shows activity averaged across 80 to 130 ms. Other time periods could be examined to address specific research questions. With respect to translating research findings to the clinic, a major hurdle will be to identify, from several data, measures that are most clinically informative. Similar to the RS

measures, this work will also involve determining whether analogous clinical findings are observed across MEG recording systems and analysis methods.

Finally, radiologists interested in this area are likely to come across a very active line of research examining the hypothesis that sensory overload and attention dysfunction in patients with Sz is due to inadequate inhibition of redundant information. In many research studies, this is experimentally demonstrated as a failure of individuals with Sz to habituate to repeated auditory stimuli.[65–67] As an example, using the "paired-click

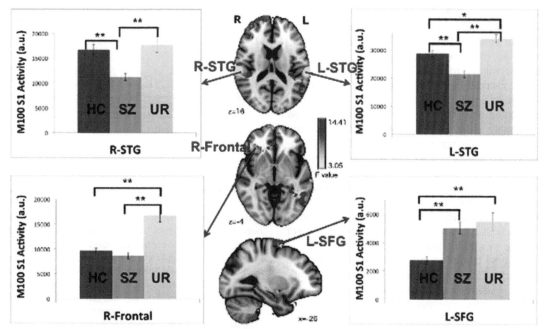

Fig. 4. Analysis of variance (ANOVA) group differences and associated bar charts showing results of 100 ms (M100) simple effects analyses at the 4 identified regions of interest (ROIs) (*P<.05, **P<.001). (*From* Chen YH, Howell B, Edgar JC. Associations and Heritability of Auditory Encoding, Gray Matter, and Attention in Schizophrenia. Schizophr Bull 2019;45(4):859-70; with permission.)

paradigm" where subjects are presented 2 clicks separated by 500 milliseconds, MEG studies compare primary/secondary auditory cortex activity with the first and second clicks in controls and individuals with Sz. MEG studies have provided mixed findings for the "gating" hypothesis, with some MEG studies showing the individuals with Sz fail to show gating/habituation to the second click (ie, a similar or larger response to the second than first click),[68] whereas other studies find no gating/habituation abnormality in Sz.[62,69] Although most studies have examined the time-domain M50 and M100 paired-click responses, other studies use time-frequency analyses to examine the frequencies associated with gating[16,70]. And although the auditory system has been the primary focus of this line of research, researchers have examined gating in the somatosensory system.[71] Finally, within this line of research, an interesting direction that will surely develop over the next decade is the use of therapy (eg, cognitive training) to normalize auditory processes in Sz.[72,73]

WHOLE-BRAIN FUNCTIONAL CONNECTIVITY MAPS

Recruitment and management of neural networks, consisting of spatially separate yet functionally related brain regions, is critical to diverse perceptual and higher-order processes. Accordingly, interest is increasing in elucidating the abnormal functional connectivity of such networks in Sz. MEG is particularly well equipped to address coordinated activity of neural networks because of its ability to measure neural oscillatory processes, its insensitivity to distortion by inhomogeneous conductivity in the head, and its excellent spatial resolution given advanced source-reconstruction algorithms and the large number of sensors now commonly used.[74–77] In addition, coregistering MEG data with high-resolution structural MR imaging improves the ability to estimate the neural generators of MEG signals by incorporating anatomic information. Findings of both hypo- and hyperconnectivity in Sz have been found across various studies using task-based and RS data, but particular patterns of connectivity may reflect specific symptoms that vary across samples.

Because disrupted information processing is a hallmark of Sz and related to a variety of symptoms, whole-brain connectivity assessed during various cognitive tasks may be clinically relevant.[78] As an example, Hirvonen and colleagues[79] found that both local and cross-region gamma-band (30–120 Hz) synchronization (a mechanism of connectivity) was lower in patients with Sz than in controls during a task requiring

perceptual integration. The functional connectivity measures were of clinical interest, with reduced gamma-band synchronization associated with more severe disorganization symptoms (**Fig. 5**). Although this image might look to some degree as a diffusion image (eg, a fractional anisotropy brain diffusion map familiar to neuroradiologists), several features of this gamma-band functional connectivity image are of note. First, the functional connectivity information (colored lines) is superimposed on an inflated and flattened cortical surface. This facilitates visualization of the connections between brain areas. Second, measures of functional connectivity were computed for regions of a priori interest. This was done to reduce the number of

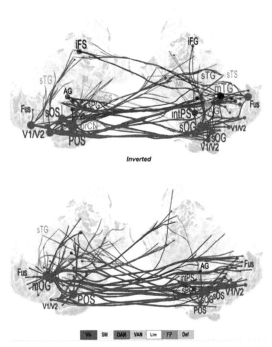

Fig. 5. Low gamma-band (30–40 Hz) cortical networks stronger for controls than Sz for upright faces (*top*) and inverted faces (*bottom*). Graphs display the 200 strongest connections on a flattened, inflated cortical surface. Red = visual network (Vis); Green = sensorimotor network (SM); Purple = dorsal attention network (DAN); Yellow = ventral attention network (VAN); Blue = frontoparietal network. AG, angular gyrus; Fus, fusiform gyrus; iFS/G, inferior frontal sulcus/gyrus; MI, primary motor cortex; mOG, middle occipital gyrus; mTG, middle temporal gyrus; POS, parieto-occipital sulcus; prCN, precuneus; SI, primary somatosensory cortex; sTG, superior temporal gyrus. (*From* Hirvonen J, Wibral M, Palva JM, et al. Whole-brain source-reconstructed MEG-data reveal reduced long-range synchronization in chronic schizophrenia. eNeuro 2017;4(5); with permission.)

calculations (from many, many thousands to tens or hundreds). Third, the functional connectivity data were scaled to show only connections with the greatest group difference (in this figure, showing the 200 most significant connections).

Research investigating RS MEG connectivity also shows abnormal network connectivity in adults with Sz.[80–83] As an example, using pairwise correlations in independent component analysis–derived RS networks across all frequency bands, Houck and colleagues[84] observed enhanced functional connectivity in frontal networks during RS in patients with Sz. **Fig. 6** shows a common way of plotting functional connectivity maps. **Fig. 6** shows connectivity results for controls (left), patients (center), and the group difference (right). The x and y axes list brain regions, with the color scale showing the significance of the connection for each pair of brain regions.

Functional connectivity methods add another layer of complexity to be considered, as the functional connectivity measures that can be computed are nearly infinite, and the clinical research literature has not settled on a standard set of measures. Studies to date primarily examine functional connectivity (amplitude or phase) within a specific frequency band (eg, connectivity between the strength of occipital gamma and frontal gamma activity). Other connectivity measures are of interest, such as phase-amplitude coupling measures that assess how the phase of low-frequency activity in one brain region modulates the strength of high-frequency activity in another brain region.[85–87] The principle is that higher-frequency activity facilitates and reflects the operation of local brain networks and that lower-frequency activity facilitates and reflects control of one region by another.[88] For example, it has been hypothesized that a failure in theta

and alpha activity modulation of gamma activity is a mechanism that fosters poor cognitive interference control in Sz. In support of this proposal, Popov and colleagues[89] reported weaker coupling of the phase of theta-band activity in anterior cingulate cortex to the amplitude of gamma-band activity in middle frontal gyrus in individuals with Sz than in healthy comparison participants.

Although relationships between disruptions in neural network dynamics and pathologic symptoms in Sz are observed in many studies using MEG recordings (as well as those using EEG and fMR imaging), findings vary across studies. This variability may correspond to methodological differences in collection and processing of MEG data as well as nosographic variability[90] in line with the growing consensus that traditional psychiatric diagnostic categories are etiologically and mechanistically diverse (eg,[31]). It may be preferable to use MEG connectivity measures to assess specific functional and symptom domains and constructs relevant to Sz, as highlighted by the Research Domain Criteria Framework.[91–93]

Despite the diversity of findings in the literature, analysis of MEG connectivity can provide important information regarding neural network dysfunction that disrupts information processing in Sz, resulting in a variety of clinical symptoms and cognitive performance deficits. Although use of MEG connectivity measures in Sz is in its infancy, it is a promising tool for elucidating the unique functional architecture of Sz, including aberrant neural integration and/or segregation, related to clinical presentation. Finally, and analogous to the RS and auditory Sz studies, functional connectivity in Sz has not yet demonstrated the degree of sensitivity and specificity that would be needed for routine clinical use.

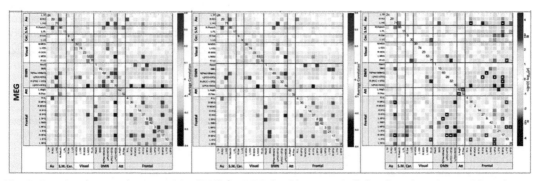

Fig. 6. Functional network connectivity (FNC) for MEG, healthy controls (left column), patients with Sz (center column), and false discovery rate corrected group differences (right column). Color scale describes the *P*-value after FDR correction. (*From* Houck JM, Cetin MS, Mayer AR. Magnetoencephalographic and functional MRI connectomics in schizophrenia via intra- and inter-network connectivity. Neuroimage 2017;145(Pt A):96-106; with permission.)

GENERAL COMMENTS AND FUTURE DIRECTIONS

MEG systems are much less common in and outside of radiology departments than are EEG and MR imaging systems and thus less available for both clinical and research use. This scarcity is a primary factor holding back clinical application of MEG, with the resulting corollary that the expert user community is small as well. As such, neither the large established base of EEG users nor the growth of fMR imaging users are pursuing the translational research needed to move MEG technology into the clinic.

Aside from the need to develop a larger user base, as detailed in this article and also Mingxiong Huang and colleagues' article, "Magnetoencephalography for Mild TBI and PTSD" in this issue, the future of clinical MEG likely depends on increased standardization and a gradual move from a qualitative to a quantitative/actuarial framework. At present, clinical MEG assessment relies primarily on careful and intensive examination of each subject's MEG data. This qualitative tradition likely reflects the development of clinical use of MEG to date principally as a tool to localize epileptiform activity (see Susan M. Bowyer and colleagues' article, "Pre-surgical Functional Mapping with Magnetoencephalography (MEG)", in this issue). In such an application, individual aspects of each clinical case (including seizure source, trade-offs of extent of surgical resection vs risk of functional loss) are critical and not yet sufficiently subject to quantitative standardization. Clinical-theoretical and actuarial approaches can be thought of as extremes on a continuum of quantification.[94] At the qualitative end are assessment approaches built on detailed observations of MEG activity, with particular weight given to human judgment about the manner in which MEG activity is abnormal, but which lack objective standardization. In contrast, actuarial systems rely on statistical evaluations of scores, derived from a standard set of protocols and analysis methods. Although at present much more emphasis on quantitative approaches is needed, Lezak[94] notes that "… to do justice to a field of inquiry as complex as brain-behavior relationships in adult human beings requires an adaptable assessment methodology that incorporates the strengths of both quantitative and qualitative approaches" (pg. 4). Because clinical judgment can be used as an input to such quantitative methods, the field is well positioned for such an integration.

For routine clinical practice, more fundamental than standardization of data-integration methods is standardization of data-acquisition methods. At present, there are few MEG clinical protocols that are standardized beyond individual centers. MEG research examination protocols vary widely as well. In addition, MEG recording systems and associated analysis algorithms vary across laboratories. For example, for auditory tasks, some laboratories use insert headphones, whereas other laboratories use free-field speakers. Even for spontaneous resting data, laboratories differ in how resting data are obtained. Similar variability is observed in data analysis procedures. Whereas some laboratories use single dipole strategies to localize auditory cortex activity, the use of whole-brain distributed source localization techniques to obtain whole-brain images is of interest and is growing, with different laboratories using different source localization routines (eg, beamforming, L1, or L2 minimum norm).

Development of new clinical indications for MEG requires a multipronged approach. This will include standardization of protocols, data collection, and data analysis procedures. Although such procedural standardization is possible and surely inevitable, some variability will remain, as MEG hardware, software, and other site-specific factors (eg, environmental electromagnetic noise levels) differ across sites. It is hoped that the gradual establishment and validation of standard presentation and analysis protocols will allow merging of data across sites and the development of normative databases. Development of normative databases in turn will foster a quantitative and generalizable approach to clinical interpretation.

ACKNOWLEDGMENTS

The authors report no conflicts of interest. This article was supported in part by NIH grant R01MH107506 (J.C. Edgar), R21MH098204 (J.C. Edgar), and R21 NS090192 (J.C. Edgar), NICHD grant R01HD093776 (J.C. Edgar), and the Intellectual and Developmental Disabilities Research Center funded by NICHD grant 5U54HD086984 (principal investigator, M. Robinson, PhD), R01 MH110544S1 (G.A. Miller).

REFERENCES

1. American Psychiatric Association. Diagnostic and statistical manual of mental disorders. 5th edition. Washington, DC: American Psychiatric Association; 2013.
2. Belbasis L, Kohler CA, Stefanis N, et al. Risk factors and peripheral biomarkers for schizophrenia spectrum disorders: an umbrella review of meta-analyses. ActaPsychiatrScand 2018;137(2):88–97.
3. Duncan LE, Keller MC. A critical review of the first 10 years of candidate gene-by-environment interaction

research in psychiatry. Am J Psychiatry 2011; 168(10):1041–9.

4. Guloksuz S, Pries LK, Delespaul P, et al. Examining the independent and joint effects of molecular genetic liability and environmental exposures in schizophrenia: results from the EUGEI study. World Psychiatry 2019;18(2):173–82.

5. Perala J, Suvisaari J, Saarni SI, et al. Lifetime prevalence of psychotic and bipolar I disorders in a general population. Arch Gen Psychiatry 2007;64(1):19–28.

6. Radua J, Ramella-Cravaro V, Ioannidis JPA, et al. What causes psychosis? An umbrella review of risk and protective factors. World Psychiatry 2018;17(1):49–66.

7. Berger GE, Bartholomeusz CF, Wood SJ, et al. Ventricular volumes across stages of schizophrenia and other psychoses. Aust N Z J Psychiatry 2017;51(10): 1041–51.

8. Pantelis C, Yucel M, Wood SJ, et al. Structural brain imaging evidence for multiple pathological processes at different stages of brain development in schizophrenia. Schizophr Bull 2005;31(3):672–96.

9. van Erp TG, Hibar DP, Rasmussen JM, et al. Subcortical brain volume abnormalities in 2028 individuals with schizophrenia and 2540 healthy controls via the ENIGMA consortium. MolPsychiatry 2016;21(4): 547–53.

10. Edgar JC, Chen YH, Lanza M, et al. Cortical thickness as a contributor to abnormal oscillations in schizophrenia? NeuroimageClin 2014;4:122–9.

11. Shenton ME, Dickey CC, Frumin M, et al. A review of MRI findings in schizophrenia. Schizophr Res 2001; 49(1–2):1–52.

12. Smiley JF, Rosoklija G, Mancevski B, et al. Altered volume and hemispheric asymmetry of the superficial cortical layers in the schizophrenia planumtemporale. Eur J Neurosci 2009;30(3):449–63.

13. Edgar JC, Fisk CL 4th, Chen YH, et al. Identifying auditory cortex encoding abnormalities in schizophrenia: The utility of low-frequency versus 40 Hz steady-state measures. Psychophysiology 2018; 55(8):e13074.

14. Grent-'t-Jong T, Rivolta D, Sauer A, et al. MEG-measured visually induced gamma-band oscillations in chronic schizophrenia: Evidence for impaired generation of rhythmic activity in ventral stream regions. Schizophr Res 2016;176(2–3):177–85.

15. Huang MX, Edgar JC, Thoma RJ, et al. Predicting EEG responses using MEG sources in superior temporal gyrus reveals source asynchrony in patients with schizophrenia. ClinNeurophysiol 2003;114(5): 835–50.

16. Popov T, Jordanov T, Weisz N, et al. Evoked and induced oscillatory activity contributes to abnormal auditory sensory gating in schizophrenia. Neuroimage 2011;56(1):307–14.

17. Rojas DC, Arciniegas DB, Teale PD, et al. Magnetoencephalography and magnetic source imaging:

technology overview and applications in psychiatric neuroimaging. CNSSpectr 1999;4(8):37–43.

18. Silverstein S, Uhlhaas PJ, Essex B, et al. Perceptual organization in first episode schizophrenia and ultra-high-risk states. Schizophr Res 2006;83(1):41–52.

19. Teale P, Reite M, Rojas DC, et al. Fine structure of the auditory M100 in schizophrenia and schizoaffective disorder. BiolPsychiatry 2000;48(11):1109–12.

20. Thune H, Recasens M, Uhlhaas PJ. The 40-Hz Auditory Steady-State Response in Patients With Schizophrenia: A Meta-analysis. JAMA Psychiatry 2016; 73(11):1145–53.

21. Wilson TW, Hernandez OO, Asherin RM, et al. Cortical gamma generators suggest abnormal auditory circuitry in early-onset psychosis. CerebCortex 2008;18(2):371–8.

22. Zeev-Wolf M, Levy J, Jahshan C, et al. MEG resting-state oscillations and their relationship to clinical symptoms in schizophrenia. NeuroimageClin 2018; 20:753–61.

23. Schizophrenia Working Group of the Psychiatric Genomics Consortium. Biological insights from 108 schizophrenia-associated genetic loci. Nature 2014;511(7510):421–7.

24. Henriksen MG, Nordgaard J, Jansson LB. Genetics of Schizophrenia: Overview of Methods, Findings and Limitations. Front Hum Neurosci 2017;11:322.

25. Dean K, Murray RM. Environmental risk factors for psychosis. DialoguesClinNeurosci 2005;7(1):69–80.

26. van Os J, Kenis G, Rutten BP. The environment and schizophrenia. Nature 2010;468(7321):203–12.

27. Andreasen NC. The evolving concept of schizophrenia: from Kraepelin to the present and future. Schizophr Res 1997;28(2–3):105–9.

28. EdgarJC, MillerGA. Identifying neural abnormalities in schizophrenia. In: Papanicolaou AC, Roberts TPL, Wheless JW, editors. Fifty years of MEG: the Oxford handbook of magnetoencephalography. Oxford University Press, in press.

29. Miller GA, Rockstroh B. Endophenotypes in psychopathology research: Where do we stand. Annu Rev ClinPsychol 2013;9:177–213.

30. Miller GA, Rockstroh B. Progress and prospects for endophenotypes for schizophrenia in the time of genomics, epigenetics, oscillatory dynamics, and RDoC. In: Nickl-Jockschat T, Abel T, editors. The neurobiology of schizophrenia. Elsevier; 2016. p. 17-38.

31. Yee CM, Javitt DC, Miller GA. Replacing DSM Categorical Analyses With Dimensional Analyses in Psychiatry Research: The Research Domain Criteria Initiative. JAMA Psychiatry 2015;72(12):1159–60.

32. Lund TR, Sponheim SR, Iacono WG, et al. Internal consistency reliability of resting EEG power spectra in schizophrenic and normal subjects. Psychophysiology 1995;32(1):66–71.

33. Canive JM, Lewine JD, Edgar JC, et al. Sponta-neous brain magnetic activity in schizophrenia patients treated with aripiprazole. Psychopharmacol Bull 1998;34(1):101–5.

34. Canive JM, Lewine JD, Edgar JC, et al. Magnetoencephalographic assessment of spontaneous brain activity in schizophrenia. Psychopharmacol Bull 1996;32(4):741–50.

35. Grent-'t-Jong T, Gross J, Goense J, et al. Resting-state gamma-band power alterations in schizophrenia reveal E/I-balance abnormalities across illness-stages. Elife 2018;7. https://doi.org/10.7554/eLife.37799.

36. Rutter L, Carver FW, Holroyd T, et al. Magnetoencephalographic gamma power reduction in patients with schizophrenia during resting condition. Hum BrainMapp 2009;30(10):3254–64.

37. Fehr T, Kissler J, Moratti S, et al. Source distribution of neuromagnetic slow waves and MEG-delta activity in schizophrenic patients. BiolPsychiatry 2001;50(2):108–16.

38. Pascual-Marqui RD, Lehmann D, Koenig T, et al. Low resolution brain electromagnetic tomography (LORETA) functional imaging in acute, neuroleptic-naive, first-episode, productive schizophrenia. Psychiatry Res 1999;90(3):169–79.

39. Rockstroh B, Watzl H, Kowalik ZJ, et al. Dynamical aspects of the EEG in different psychopathological states in an interview situation: a pilot study. Schizophr Res 1997;28(1):77–85.

40. Sponheim SR, Clementz BA, Iacono WG, et al. Resting EEG in first-episode and chronic schizophrenia. Psychophysiology 1994;31(1):37–43.

41. Weinberger DR. Schizophrenia and the frontal lobe. TrendsNeurosci 1988;11(8):367–70.

42. Wienbruch C, Moratti S, Elbert T, et al. Source distribution of neuromagnetic slow wave activity in schizophrenic and depressive patients. ClinNeurophysiol 2003;114(11):2052–60.

43. Winterer G, Ziller M, Dorn H, et al. Frontal dysfunction in schizophrenia–a new electrophysiological classifier for research and clinical applications. Eur Arch PsychiatryClinNeurosci 2000;250(4):207–14.

44. Galderisi S, Mucci A, Volpe U, et al. Evidence-based medicine and electrophysiology in schizophrenia. ClinEEGNeurosci 2009;40:62–77.

45. Lisman J. Excitation, inhibition, local oscillations, or large-scale loops: what causes the symptoms of schizophrenia? CurrOpinNeurobiol 2012;22(3):537–44.

46. Llinas R, Urbano FJ, Leznik E, et al. Rhythmic and dysrhythmicthalamocortical dynamics: GABA systems and the edge effect. TrendsNeurosci 2005;28(6):325–33.

47. Huang MX, Nichols S, Robb A, et al. An automatic MEG low-frequency source imaging approach for detecting injuries in mild and moderate TBI patients with blast and non-blast causes. Neuroimage 2012;61(4):1067–82.

48. Huang MX, Theilmann RJ, Robb A, et al. Integrated imaging approach with MEG and DTI to detect mild traumatic brain injury in military and civilian patients. J Neurotrauma 2009;26(8):1213–26.

49. Chen YH, Stone-Howell B, Edgar JC, et al. Frontal slow-wave activity as a predictor of negative symptoms, cognition and functional capacity in schizophrenia. Br J Psychiatry 2016;208(2):160–7.

50. Lewine JD, Orrison WW. Chapter 9 - Magnetoencephalography and Magnetic Source Imaging. In: Orrison WW, Lewine JD, Sanders JA, et al, editors. Functional Brain Imaging. St Louis: Mosby Yearbooks; 1995. p. 369-417.

51. Rockstroh BS, Wienbruch C, Ray WJ, et al. Abnormal oscillatory brain dynamics in schizophrenia: a sign of deviant communication in neural network? BMC Psychiatry 2007;7:44.

52. Edgar JC, Dipiero M, McBride E, et al. Abnormal maturation of the resting-state peak alpha frequency in children with autism spectrum disorder. Hum BrainMapp 2019. https://doi.org/10.1002/hbm.24598.

53. Miskovic V, Ma X, Chou CA, et al. Developmental changes in spontaneous electrocortical activity and network organization from early to late childhood. Neuroimage 2015;118:237–47.

54. Somsen RJ, van'tKlooster BJ, van der Molen MW, et al. Growth spurts in brain maturation during middle childhood as indexed by EEG power spectra. BiolPsychol 1997;44(3):187–209.

55. Szava S, Valdes P, Biscay R, et al. High resolution quantitative EEG analysis. Brain Topogr 1994;6(3):211–9.

56. Valdes P, Valdes M, Carballo JA, et al. QEEG in a public health system. Brain Topogr 1992;4(4):259–66.

57. Chen YH, Howell B, Edgar JC, et al. Associations and Heritability of Auditory Encoding, Gray Matter, and Attention in Schizophrenia. Schizophr Bull 2018. https://doi.org/10.1093/schbul/sby111.

58. Greenwood TA, Braff DL, Light GA, et al. Initial heritability analyses of endophenotypic measures for schizophrenia: the consortium on the genetics of schizophrenia. Arch Gen Psychiatry 2007;64(11):1242–50.

59. Kustermann T, Rockstroh B, Kienle J, et al. Deficient attention modulation of lateralized alpha power in schizophrenia. Psychophysiology 2016;53(6):776–85.

60. Rosburg T, Boutros NN, Ford JM. Reduced auditory evoked potential component N100 in schizophrenia–a critical review. Psychiatry Res 2008;161(3):259–74.

61. Schubring D, Popov T, Miller GA, et al. Consistency of abnormal sensory gating in first-admission and chronic schizophrenia across quantification

methods. Psychophysiology 2018;55(4). https://doi.org/10.1111/psyp.13006.

62. Smith AK, Edgar JC, Huang M, et al. Cognitive abilities and 50- and 100-msec paired-click processes in schizophrenia. Am J Psychiatry 2010;167(10):1264–75.

63. Turetsky BI, Greenwood TA, Olincy A, et al. Abnormal auditory N100 amplitude: a heritable endophenotype in first-degree relatives of schizophrenia probands. BiolPsychiatry 2008;64(12):1051–9.

64. Edgar JC, Huang MX, Weisend MP, et al. Interpreting abnormality: an EEG and MEG study of P50 and the auditory paired-stimulus paradigm. BiolPsychol 2003;65(1):1–20.

65. Adler LE, Pachtman E, Franks RD, et al. Neurophysiological evidence for a defect in neuronal mechanisms involved in sensory gating in schizophrenia. BiolPsychiatry 1982;17(6):639–54.

66. Braff DL. Information processing and attention dysfunctions in schizophrenia. Schizophr Bull 1993;19(2):233–59.

67. Yee CM, Nuechterlein KH, Morris SE, et al. P50 suppression in recent-onset schizophrenia: clinical correlates and risperidone effects. J AbnormPsychol 1998;107(4):691–8.

68. Thoma RJ, Hanlon FM, Moses SN, et al. Lateralization of auditory sensory gating and neuropsychological dysfunction in schizophrenia. Am J Psychiatry 2003;160(9):1595–605.

69. Bachmann S, Weisbrod M, Rohrig M, et al. MEG does not reveal impaired sensory gating in first-episode schizophrenia. Schizophr Res 2010;121(1–3):131–8.

70. Edgar JC, Hanlon FM, Huang MX, et al. Superior temporal gyrus spectral abnormalities in schizophrenia. Psychophysiology 2008;45(5):812–24.

71. Edgar JC, Miller GA, Moses SN, et al. Cross-modal generality of the gating deficit. Psychophysiology 2005;42(3):318–27.

72. Popov T, Rockstroh B, Weisz N, et al. Adjusting brain dynamics in schizophrenia by means of perceptual and cognitive training. PLoS One 2012;7(7):e39051.

73. Popova P, Rockstroh B, Miller GA, et al. The impact of cognitive training on spontaneous gamma oscillations in schizophrenia. Psychophysiology 2018;55(8):e13083.

74. Brookes MJ, Hale JR, Zumer JM, et al. Measuring functional connectivity using MEG: methodology and comparison with fcMRI. Neuroimage 2011;56(3):1082–104.

75. Cohen D. Magnetoencephalography: detection of the brain's electrical activity with a superconducting magnetometer. Science 1972;175(4022):664–6.

76. Schoffelen JM, Gross J. Source connectivity analysis with MEG and EEG. Hum BrainMapp 2009;30(6):1857–65.

77. Zumer JM, Attias HT, Sekihara K, et al. A probabilistic algorithm integrating source localization and noise suppression for MEG and EEG data. Neuroimage 2007;37(1):102–15.

78. Ioannides AA, Poghosyan V, Dammers J, et al. Real-time neural activity and connectivity in healthy individuals and schizophrenia patients. Neuroimage 2004;23(2):473–82.

79. Hirvonen J, Wibral M, Palva JM, et al. Whole-brain source-reconstructed MEG-data reveal reduced long-range synchronization in chronic schizophrenia. eNeuro 2017;4(5). https://doi.org/10.1523/ENEURO.0338-17.2017.

80. Cetin MS, Houck JM, Rashid B, et al. Multimodal Classification of Schizophrenia Patients with MEG and fMRI Data Using Static and Dynamic Connectivity Measures. Front Neurosci 2016;10:466.

81. Hinkley LB, Vinogradov S, Guggisberg AG, et al. Clinical symptoms and alpha band resting-state functional connectivity imaging in patients with schizophrenia: implications for novel approaches to treatment. BiolPsychiatry 2011;70(12):1134–42.

82. Robinson SE, Mandell AJ. Mutual Information in a MEG complexity measure suggests regional hyper-connectivity in schizophrenic probands. Neuropsychopharmacology 2015;40(1):251–2.

83. Rutter L, Nadar SR, Holroyd T, et al. Graph theoretical analysis of resting magnetoencephalographic functional connectivity networks. Front ComputNeurosci 2013;7:93.

84. Houck JM, Cetin MS, Mayer AR, et al. Magnetoencephalographic and functional MRI connectomics in schizophrenia via intra- and inter-network connectivity. Neuroimage 2017;145(Pt A):96–106.

85. Berman JI, McDaniel J, Liu S, et al. Variable bandwidth filtering for improved sensitivity of cross-frequency coupling metrics. Brain Connect 2012;2(3):155–63.

86. Canolty RT, Edwards E, Dalal SS, et al. High gamma power is phase-locked to theta oscillations in human neocortex. Science 2006;313(5793):1626–8.

87. Osipova D, Hermes D, Jensen O. Gamma power is phase-locked to posterior alpha activity. PLoS One 2008;3(12):e3990.

88. Canolty RT, Knight RT. The functional role of cross-frequency coupling. TrendsCognSci 2010;14(11):506–15.

89. Popov T, Wienbruch C, Meissner S, et al. A mechanism of deficient interregional neural communication in schizophrenia. Psychophysiology 2015;52(5):648–56.

90. Alamian G, Hincapie AS, Pascarella A, et al. Measuring alterations in oscillatory brain networks in schizophrenia with resting-state MEG: State-of-the-art and methodological challenges. ClinNeurophysiol 2017;128(9):1719–36.

91. Kozak MJ, Cuthbert BN. The NIMH research domain criteria initiative: background, issues, and pragmatics. Psychophysiology 2016;53(3):286–97.

92. Lake JI, Yee CM, Miller GA. Misunderstanding RDoC. ZietschriftPsychol 2017;225(3):170–4.

93. Miller GA. Comments on Kendler's "The Impact of Faculty Psychology and Theories of Psychological Causation on the Origins of Modern Psychiatric Nosology". In: Kendler KS, Parnas J, Zachar P, editors. Levels of analysis in psychopathology: Cross-disciplinary perspectives. New York: Cambridge University Press; 2020. p. 479-90.

94. Lezak MD. Neuropsychological assessment. New York: Oxford University Press; 1995.

Role of Magnetoencephalography in the Early Stages of Alzheimer Disease

Fernando Maestú, PhD[a,b,*], Alberto Fernández, PhD[b,c]

KEYWORDS

- Magnetoencephalography • Mild cognitive impairment • Preclinical stages • Prodromal stages
- Functional connectivity • Power • Alzheimer disease

KEY POINTS

- Alzheimer disease (AD) can be understood now as a continuum where mild cognitive impairment (MCI), is one of the key stages.
- The most frequently used AD biomarkers are devoted to the detection of Aβ deposition and tau pathology by means of cerebrospinal fluid analysis or PET imaging (ie, PET-amyloid or PET-tau).
- The role of electroencephalography and magnetoencephalography in the diagnosis and investigation of the AD-continuum is growing and better defined.

INTRODUCTION TO ALZHEIMER DISEASE

Alzheimer disease (AD) is the most common cause of dementing illness around the world and comprises 60% of all dementia cases.[1] The risk of developing AD increases with age. This is a crucial issue considering the tendency to older populations in the western countries, and consequently AD became one of the main health challenges of our societies. From a neurobiological perspective, AD is characterized by the accumulation of amyloid-beta (Aβ) protein, the hyperphosphorylation of tau protein and neuroinflammation. These pathologic processes are believed to lead to a synaptic dysfunction/neurodegeneration and finally to neural death and severe cognitive deterioration. A closely related concept, now involved in the so-called AD-continuum, is mild cognitive impairment (MCI). MCI was a term initially used to describe the transitional state between a healthy cognitive status and dementia. Patients with a diagnosis of MCI were considered at a higher risk of developing AD, with a much higher conversion rate to dementia when compared with healthy controls.[2] With the progression of research, it appeared more and more clear that MCI was a too unspecific concept, with subjects showing different courses, including the reversion to a cognitively "normal" condition. Recent diagnosis criteria stressed the importance of a correct detection of the actual underlying pathology that is producing the cognitive manifestations, leading to concepts such as "MCI due to AD" or "prodromal AD."[3,4] The detection of these prodromal or predementia cases is essential, and the electrophysiological techniques demonstrated a notable performance (see later in this article).

Currently, the most frequently used AD biomarkers are devoted to the detection of Aβ deposition and tau pathology by means of

[a] Department of Experimental Psychology, Complutense University of Madrid, Madrid, Spain; [b] Centro de Tecnología Biomédica, Campus de Montegancedo de la UPM, Pozuelo de Alarcón, Madrid 28223, Spain; [c] Department of Legal Medicine, Psychiatry and Pathology, Complutense University of Madrid, Madrid, Spain
* Corresponding author. Centro de Tecnología Biomédica, Campus de Montegancedo de la UPM, Pozuelo de Alarcón, Madrid 28223, Spain.
E-mail address: fmaestuu@ucm.es

Neuroimag Clin N Am 30 (2020) 217–227
https://doi.org/10.1016/j.nic.2020.01.003
1052-5149/20/Published by Elsevier Inc.

cerebrospinal fluid (CSF) analysis or PET imaging (ie, PET-amyloid or PET-tau). PET with fluorodeoxyglucose is considered a marker of synaptic dysfunction, whereas MR imaging volumetry is the most common measure of atrophy (for a full perspective on these issues see Refs.[5–7]). Other techniques might allow an additional assessment of some of these basic pathologic changes. As previously noted, synaptic dysfunction is one of the earliest manifestations of AD pathology. In this regard, electroencephalography (EEG) and magnetoencephalography (MEG) are capable of detecting the synchronized oscillatory activity of thousands of neurons that relies on the integrity of neural connections. Moreover, both techniques measure neural activity directly and with millisecond temporal resolution.[8] Despite these clear advantages, the role of EEG and MEG in the diagnosis and investigation of the AD-continuum is not well defined. As Stam[9] pointed out in his excellent review on the role of EEG in dementias, some investigators claimed that such a role may be limited to exclude rare neurologic conditions. On the contrary, Winblad and colleagues[10] suggested that a relevant focus of AD/MCI research should be the development of guidelines for neurophysiological evaluation techniques, as they are cheaper and totally noninvasive compared with CSF or PET-derived biomarkers, whereas their sensitivity is very similar.[9] In the next pages we present some of the evidence that may support the affirmation of Winblad and colleagues.[10]

ELECTROPHYSIOLOGICAL CORRELATES IN THE ALZHEIMER DISEASE SPECTRUM

The "abnormalities" of EEGs of patients with AD were first described by Hans Berger.[11,12] After a century of EEG investigations, the pattern of resting-state brain electrical activity in AD has been characterized in terms of a gradual and relatively diffuse "slowing." Overall, the literature on spectral measures revealed a progressive increase of the absolute and relative power in delta and theta bands and a power decrease in alpha and beta within patients with AD, usually focused in the temporoparietal and occipital regions.[13–16] Perhaps one of the most straightforward procedures to perceive this pattern of slowing is the calculation of the alpha peak frequency. A slowing of the alpha peak (typical range 8–13 Hz) has been observed in normal aging.[17] The alpha peaks in patients with AD exhibit a more pronounced "shift to the left," sometimes interpreted as support for the hypothesis of an accelerated aging process. In fact, abnormally low alpha peak frequencies are usually described in patients with AD.[18] In addition, the sources of alpha activity may move to a more frontal localization, the so-called "frontalization" of alpha, and such shift to anterior regions seems to correlate with the severity of the disease.[19] Of note, subjects with MCI tend to show an intermediate situation between patients with AD and healthy controls in the previously described measures.

This evidence may be solidly based on 2 physiologic determinants that could explain the slowing of brain electrical activity in AD. The first candidate is a cholinergic deficit. Some classic studies[20,21] reported a significant correlation between loss of cholinergic neurons, reduced acetylcholinesterase levels, and delta power in patients with AD. This correlation was experimentally supported in animal and human models by the administration of scopolamine (a cholinergic antagonist) infusions that generated an increased delta and theta power.[22] However, some other investigations revealed that a more widespread neurodegenerative process involving cholinergic, monoaminergic, glutamatergic, and even other neurotransmitter systems are necessary to produce the frequency slowing.[23] A complementary hypothesis relies on the notion that AD can be considered a disconnection syndrome.[24] It is well-known that corticothalamic deafferentation and white-matter lesions produce a typical pattern of polymorphic delta activity described by Gloor and coworkers.[25] Holschneider and Leuchter[26] claimed that such a disconnection syndrome could play a role not only in the increased delta activity but also in the decreased beta activity observed in AD.

Following this reasoning thread, it is not surprising that the brain activity slowing in AD correlates with other manifestations of the disease, such as cortical and hippocampal atrophy (signs of neurodegeneration) or cognitive performance.[27,28] From a genetic perspective, Lehtovirta and colleagues[29,30] described an extra slowing of the EEG spectrum in patients with AD carrying the APOE4 allele, in comparison with noncarriers, that was explained by the influence of APOE on cholinergic neuron functioning.

MAGNETOENCEPHALOGRAPHY CORRELATES OF ALZHEIMER DISEASE

Similar to EEG, MEG is a noninvasive technique that offers a direct measure of neural activity. MEG is a young technique as compared with EEG, and its application to the AD-continuum has been relatively recent. In fact, the first papers devoted to the investigation of AD by means of MEG appeared in the late 1990s.[31,32] In the forthcoming pages it will be shown that most of the previously described EEG evidence of electro-physiological changes in AD have been replicated by MEG studies. Notwithstanding, it is important to bear in mind that MEG has some technical features due to physical properties of the magnetic fields, such as the more accurate source reconstruction and the sensitivity to a broader frequency spectrum, that offer an important advantage as compared with EEG. In this section, the studies of spectral variations observed in AD and its prodromal stages (both in sensor and source space), as well as functional networks research are reviewed. Of particular interest are the follow-up studies investigating MEG markers of progression to AD.

Resting-State Magnetoencephalography Spectral Analysis

As previously noted, MEG studies virtually mirrored the results obtained by EEG. Berendse and coworkers[33] demonstrated in early investigations that brain activity slowing was also reproduced in MEG recordings. When an exhaustive frequency analysis was accomplished, the relative power in 2 intervals (2–4 Hz and 16–28 Hz) allowed a correct classification of healthy controls and AD cases.[34,35] In addition, mean frequency analysis also supported a progressive slowing, not only in patients with AD but also in MCIs, with the latter group exhibiting an intermediate position between ADs and controls[34,35] (Table 1). This study confirmed the progressive "shift to the left" of the dominant alpha activity with the progress of the disease. Interestingly, when the MCI subtype was considered, the amnestic multidomain cases showed increased delta and theta power as compared with the single-domain cases, thus indicating that brain activity slowing in multidomain MCI resembled the typical pattern observed in AD.[36]

All the preceding MEG studies were performed in the sensor space. However, as was previously stressed, MEG offers a clear advantage in terms of source localization as compared with EEG. In this vein, Fernández and coworkers[37] performed the first MEG source localization of delta and theta activity in AD, demonstrating a significant increase within temporoparietal regions that correlated with cognitive status. Mirroring EEG, that temporoparietal low-frequency activity correlated with hippocampal atrophy, but more importantly, a combination of MEG and volumetric data allowed the correct classification of 87.1% of patients with AD vs controls.[38] Osipova and coworkers[39,40] confirmed that alpha sources in posterior brain regions were substituted by lower frequencies in

ADs but the evidence was not reproduced in MCI cases. Engels and coworkers[41] showed that the pattern of slowing observed in AD was present not only at the cortical level but also in the hippocampus, as evidenced by means of the utilization of virtual electrodes.

Recently, this line of research has been extended to earlier stages, such as subjective cognitive decline (SCD). It is well-known that SCD increases the risk for developing dementia; however, this population cannot be considered as having any memory problem because patients perform within the average on standard neuropsychological tests. It was of great interest to see whether that "average" behavioral performance was accompanied by some type of differential feature at the neurophysiological level. López-Sanz and colleagues[42] showed how patients with SCD exhibited a decreased alpha power over bilateral prefrontal areas, bilateral middle and superior temporal lobe, and also bilaterally over calcarine fissure and cuneus in the occipital lobe. In a subsequent study, López-Sanz and colleagues[43] scanned with MEG 252 older adults (70 healthy controls, 91 SCD, and 91 MCI). Alpha relative power in the source space was used to train a LASSO classifier and applied to distinguish between healthy controls, and SCD and MCI patients. The reduction of the alpha band power was able to classify subjects with SCD with an area under the curve (AUC) of 0.81. When unseen data were classified, the AUC went to 0.75, which is still a high rate for blind approaches.

Functional Network Disruption in the Disease Process

Amyloid deposition may have a toxic effect on inhibitory terminals,[45] impairing the normal balance between excitation and inhibition of neuronal activity, increasing neuronal excitability and damaging neural network function.[46–48] Tau deposition disrupts axonal microtubule organization[49] and its deposits correlate with cognitive impairment[50] and network dysfunction.[51] This progressive loss of synaptic efficiency disrupts interregional and intraregional communication, leading to the proposal that AD is a disconnection syndrome.[52,53] Pathologic changes associated with AD, such as amyloid deposition, start decades before the first clinical symptoms appear, and most clinically relevant functional loss is thus far irrecoverable once the disease process has gone unchecked. Therefore, this depletion of the inhibitory activity could lead to increased brain activity not associated with better cognitive function.[54]

Table 1
MEG studies in preclinical AD and MCI

Author	Comparison	Sample Size	Methodology	Result
Bajo et al,[59] 2010	MCI vs CN	22 MCI, 19 CN	Sensors, Task, MEG, FC	Increased long-distance interhemispheric FC and decreased anteroposterior FC.
Buldú et al,[56] 2011	MCI vs CN	19 MCI, 19 CN	Sensors, Task, MEG, Graphs	Increased network strength and outreach.
Cuesta et al,[69] 2015	MCI vs CN f(ApoE)	20 MCIε4−, 16 MCIε4+, 8 CNε4+, 19 CNε4−	Sources, Resting, MEG, FC	Decreased alpha and beta hippocampal and IPL FC in MCI. Decreased delta FC in ApoE34. Dual increased/decreased FC pattern affecting frontal/temporal regions.
Cuesta et al,[70] 2015	MCI vs CN f(ApoE)	20 MCIε4−, 16 MCIε4+, 6 CNε4+, 19 CNε4-	Sources, Resting, MEG, Power	Increased theta power in CN ApoE34, and extra slowing in MCI Apoe34.
Fernández et al,[35] 2006	AD vs MCI vs CN	22 AD, 22 MCI, 21 CN	Sources, Resting, MEG, Median frequency	Slowing of the mean frequency with the progression of the disease. MCI intermediate position between AD and CN.
López et al,[36] 2014	MCI subtypes vs CN	33 a-sd-MCI, 36 a-md-MCI, 36 CN	Sources, Resting, MEG, Power	Low-frequency increase in both MCI groups. The a-md-MCI group showed an extra slowing that correlated with cognitive status.
López-Sanz et al,[42] 2016	MCI vs SCD vs CN	51 MCI, 41 SCD, 39 CN	Sources, Resting, MEG, Power	Decreased alpha power. MCI showed slowing in their alpha peak.
López-Sanz et al,[43] 2017	MCI vs SCD vs CN	51 MCI, 41 SCD, 39 CN	Sources, Resting, MEG, FC	Increased alpha anterior FC and decreased posterior alpha FC.
López-Sanz et al,[44] 2017	MCI vs SCD vs CN	69 MCI, 55 SCD, 63 CN	Sources, Resting, MEG, Graphs	SCD showed an intermediate degree of network disruption in multiple parameters.
Maestú et al,[54] 2008	MCI vs CN	15 MCI, 20 CN	Sources, Task, MEG, Activation	Bilateral higher activity in the ventral pathway.
Maestú et at,[57] 2015	MCI vs CN	102 MCI, 82 CN	Sensors, Resting, MEG, FC	Enhanced fronto-parietal and interhemispheric broadband FC.
Nakamura et al,[65] 2017	CNp vs CN	13 CNp, 32 CN	Sources, Resting, MEG, FC	Decreased local FC in Pcu. Increased FC between Pcu and both IPL.

(*continued on next page*)

Table 1
(continued)

Author	Comparison	Sample Size	Methodology	Result
Nakamura et al,[66] 2018	MCI vs CNp vs CN	28 MCI, 11 MCInoAD, 13 CNp, 17 CN	Sources, Resting, MEG, Power	Increased frontal alpha power in MCI and CNp. Increased frontal delta power in MCI vs CNp. Global increased theta power in MCI.
Osipova et al,[40] 2006	AD vs MCI vs CN	11 AD, 9 MCI, 10 CN	Sources, Resting, MEG, Power	Alpha slowing and anteriorization in AD, no differences in MCI group.

Abbreviations: AD, Alzheimer's disease; a-md-MCI, amnestic multidomain MCI; a-sd-MCI, amnestic single-domain MCI; CN, control; CNp, controls amyloid positive; FC, functional connectivity; IPL, inferior parietal lobule; MCI, mild cognitive impairment; MEG, magnetoencephalography; Pcu, precuneus; SCD, subjective cognitive decline; ε4, APOE4 carrier.

This synaptic dysfunction and disruption of local and long-distance connectivity can be studied with MEG. MEG provides a direct measure of neuronal field potentials that can be used to assess the organization of brain functional architecture in AD.[55]

Functional Network Disruption at Different Stages of the Disease

Although the dementia stage of AD may be associated with functional disconnection,[55] earlier stages also may be associated with communication disruption.[56] Indeed, MEG studies of patients with MCI found alterations in network organization across the cortex preceding clinical dementia.[57,58] In the past 20 years, the research in this field has been very active in evaluating the utility of resting-state MEG functional connectivity (MEGfc) as a biomarker of synaptic dysfunction in the early stages of AD. Resting-state functional connectivity analysis has shown a dual pattern of increasing and decreasing functional connectivity over prefrontal and posterior regions, respectively[43,54,59] (**Fig. 1**). To explore in more detail whether hypersynchronization could be a hallmark of network disruption, some MEG groups across the world joined in an international consortium (5 countries and 3 different continents). This study evaluated MEG functional networks as a biomarker at the individual level in a blind design and provided an accurate classification between MCI and controls of more than 80%.[57] Again, increased synchronization between anterior and posterior regions provided the best classification rate. However, MEGfc should be compared with current biomarkers, such as CSF or PET measures of tau and amyloid-beta.

Magnetoencephalography as a Biomarker for Conversion from Mild Cognitive Impairment to Dementia

A crucial factor for considering MEG as a biomarker for AD is its capability to predict conversion across the different stages of the disease (preclinical-prodromal-dementia). There are very few longitudinal studies, and all focused on the conversion from MCI to dementia. For example, Fernández and colleagues[60] (**Table 2**) demonstrated that the estimated relative risk of conversion to AD was increased by 350% in those MCI cases with high delta activity in left posterior parietal region. In subsequent investigations using more sensitive localization algorithms, an augmented delta activity in posterior parietal and precuneus cortices was involved in the transition from MCI to mild, and from mild to more severe dementia.[61] A recent follow-up study established that the combination of left hippocampal volume, occipital cortex theta power, and clock drawing copy subtest scores predicted conversion to AD with 100% sensitivity and 94.7% specificity.[62] This evidence supported the idea that source analysis of MEG spectral changes might be a serious candidate to reflect disease progression within the AD-continuum. Profiles of conversion from healthy subjects to MCI also were described in the context of a memory task in which medial temporal lobe number of sources was reduced in converters versus nonconverters during a memory task.

From a functional connectivity perspective, 3 longitudinal studies (2 years of follow-up) with a similar sample demonstrated that those patients with MCI who developed dementia showed higher alpha band synchronization than those who remained stable.[58,63] The higher the synchronization between the anterior cingulate cortex and the posterior

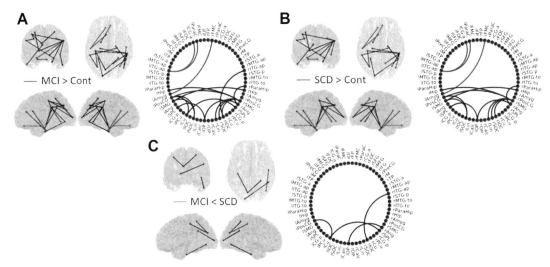

Fig. 1. Depicted are the functional connectivity differences among healthy controls, SCD, and patients with MCI. Coronal, sagittal, and axial views of MR imaging with hypersynchronized (*red*) and hyposynchronized (*blue*) links. Also represented are circle plots showing schematic views of the significant links. (*A*) The increased connectivity of the MCI group in comparison with controls in red and decreased in blue. (*B*) Increased connectivity in red in favor of SCD compared with controls and in blue, decreased connectivity. (*C*) Decreased connectivity of the subjects with MCI compared with SCD. (*Adapted from* López-Sanz D, Bruña R, Garcés P, et al. Functional Connectivity Disruption in Subjective Cognitive Decline and Mild Cognitive Impairment: A Common Pattern of Alterations. Front Aging Neurosci. 2017;9:109; with permission.)

cortical regions, the higher the likelihood for developing dementia.[58,63] Furthermore, patients who showed high levels of p-tau in the CSF and later developed dementia showed again an increased synchronization between the medial temporal lobe and the anterior cingulate cortex in the beta frequency band.[64]

Magnetoencephalography and Alzheimer Disease Biomarkers

To confirm the role of MEG as a diagnostic tool in the actual clinical scenario, it is crucial to compare its results with the current biomarkers of the disease. For instance, healthy elders without hypometabolism or brain atrophy, but with a positive amyloid burden, showed a hypersynchronization in posterior networks of the brain in comparison with amyloid-negative subjects. These profiles were directly associated with local amyloid deposition.[65,66] Canuet and coworkers[64] reported significant correlations between the levels of the p-tau protein and the functional connectivity values between medial temporal lobe and anterior cingulate cortex in subjects with prodromal AD. This finding agrees with the tau neuropathology network model as described by Braak and Braak,[67] and with recent ideas of "transneuronal neurodegeneration."[68] The potential network alterations driven by transneuronal degeneration shape a unique framework to assess, with MEG

and tau-PET, the cascade of neuropathological changes underlying AD progression. Unfortunately, this comparison has not yet been done.

A very recent paper[66] offered a new perspective on the role of MEG spectral analysis in the AD-continuum (**Fig. 2**). Patients with MCI and control subjects were evaluated and classified according to the level of amyloid burden in Aβ-positive and Aβ-negative cases. Results indicated 2 clear effects. The first one was associated with Aβ positivity and consisted of a frontalization of alpha activity that, importantly, was not correlated with cognitive status. The second one consisted of a significant increase of occipital and frontal delta that was associated with the transition from control to MCI status in the Aβ-positive cases, and consequently was considered a specific marker within the AD-continuum. This delta increase correlated with cognitive status and with 2 classic synaptic dysfunction/neurodegeneration markers, such as entorhinal atrophy and hypometabolism in posterior cingulate/precuneus. Perhaps the most intriguing finding of the study was evidence that the typically generalized theta power increase that has been considered a key electrophysiological marker of AD was not specific for the disease, as it appeared in Aβ-negative cases. Theta increase was rather a nonspecific marker of cognitive deterioration that correlated with hippocampal atrophy.

Table 2
MEG studies on the progression along AD-continuum

Author	Comparison	Sample Size	Methodology	Result
Bajo et al,[63] 2012	pMCI vs sMCI	5 pMCI, 14 sMCI	Sensors, Task, MEG, FC	Increased parieto-occipital and frontal FC.
Canuet et al,[64] 2015	pMCI vs sMCI	3 pMCI, 9 sMCI	Sources, Resting, MEG, functional connectivity	Increased beta band between hippocampus and anterior cingulate cortex, in correlation with increased tau-CSF.
Fernández et al,[60] 2006	pMCI vs sMCI	17 MCI, 17 controls	Sources, Resting, MEG, DeltaPower	Increased parietal low-frequency increases by 350% the relative risk of progressing to AD.
Fernández et al,[61] 2013	AD vs MCI vs CN	35 AD, 23 MCI, 24 CN	Sources, Resting, MEG, DeltaPower	Increased delta power in posterior parietal and precuneus indexed the transition from MCI to mild AD. Significant correlation between delta power and cognitive status.
López et al,[58] 2014	pMCI vs sMCI	19 pMCI, 30 sMCI	Sources, Resting, MEG, FC	Increased alpha FC between right anterior cingulate and temporo-occipital regions.
López et al,[62] 2016	pMCI vs sMCI	12 pMCI, 21 sMCI	Sources, Resting, MEG, DeltaPower	A combination of hippocampal volume, occipital theta power and cognitive scores classifies pMCI and sMCI with 100% sensitivity and 94.7% specificity.

Abbreviations: AD, Alzheimer's disease; CN, control; CSF, cerebrospinal fluid; FC, functional connectivity; MCI, mild cognitive impairment; MEG, magnetoencephalography; pMCI, progressive MCI; sMCI, stable MCI.

Finally, genetic factors, such as APOE-carriage, also play a modulatory role on functional networks, and healthy elders carrying the APOE-ε4 allele showed an increased synchronization[69] and a theta power augmentation in anterior regions of the brain.[70] A common factor discovered in the connectivity research was an increased synchronization between brain regions, reflecting a lack of balance between inhibition/excitation and leading to spurious synchrony. One question about these findings could be the reproducibility of the functional network results. Garcés and colleagues[71] published a study in which subjects underwent 3 MEG scans in the same day (morning time) of 3 separate weeks and the intraclass correlation was very high for phase synchrony metrics. This allows the use of the functional network approach as a monitor for future studies involving pharmacologic or nonpharmacological interventions.

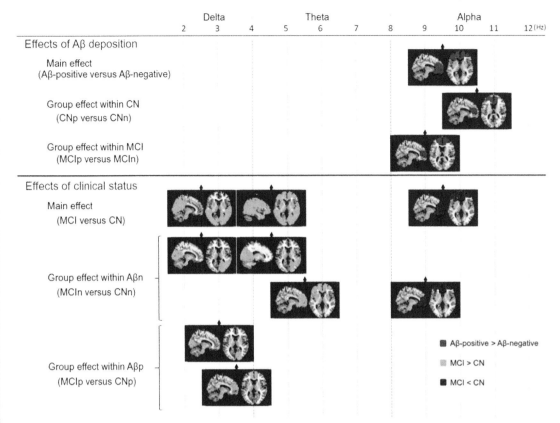

Fig. 2. MEG power markers representing the effects of amyloid-β deposits and clinical status. Each arrow indicates the peak frequency where the maximum effect was detected. The red color indicates that the amyloid-β–positive groups showed greater power than the amyloid-β–negative groups. The green colors indicate larger power in the MCI groups than a healthy control group, and the blue color indicates the opposite. CN, control; n, negative; p, positive.

SUMMARY

All of the literature reviewed in this article demonstrated that MEG is an excellent candidate biomarker for the AD-continuum. The ability of MEG to describe the patterns of synaptic disruption in the transitions from the preclinical to prodromal and dementia stages, allows its potential utilization as a diagnosis as well as a prognosis tool. The fact that a multicenter blind study provided high classification rates, using a nonhypothesis-guided approach of analysis (machine learning), demonstrated its potential for helping in the diagnosis process at the individual level.

Although all previous information supports the role of MEG as a biomarker, 3 main issues still hinder its use in the clinical scenario: (1) the presence of MEG devices in clinical facilities worldwide is still not as common as MR imaging or EEG, suggesting that MEG knowledge needs to be replicated with EEG; and (2) the correlation of MEG with current biomarkers has not been extensively evaluated yet. The investigation of how protein deposition alters the electromagnetic patterns may help to further understand the neuropathology of AD and other amyloidopathies, tauopathies, or synucleinopathies, such as Parkinson disease dementia and fronto-temporal dementia. (3) A class I prospective study in a multicenter setting is still missing. MEG manufacturers should convene to join forces and support such a study to definitively establish this new clinical application for MEG.

ACKNOWLEDGMENTS

This study was supported by two projects from the Spanish Ministry of science (PSI2012-38375-C03-01; RTI2018-098762-B-C31) and the Madrid Neurocenter (B2017/BMD-3760).

REFERENCES

1. Qiu C, Kivipelto M, von Strauss E. Epidemiology of Alzheimer's disease: occurrence, determinants,

and strategies toward intervention. Dialogues Clin Neurosci 2009;11(2):111–28.

2. Petersen RC. Mild cognitive impairment as a diagnostic entity. J Intern Med 2004;256(3):183–94.

3. Albert MS, DeKosky ST, Dickson D, et al. The diagnosis of mild cognitive impairment due to Alzheimer's disease: recommendations from the National Institute on Aging-Alzheimer's Association workgroups on diagnostic guidelines for Alzheimer's disease. Alzheimers Dement 2011;7(3):270–9.

4. Dubois B, Hampel H, Feldman HH, et al. Preclinical Alzheimer's disease: definition, natural history, and diagnostic criteria. Alzheimers Dement 2016;12(3): 292–323.

5. Dubois B, Feldman HH, Jacova C, et al. Advancing research diagnostic criteria for Alzheimer's disease: the IWG-2 criteria. Lancet Neurol 2014;13(6):614–29.

6. Dubois B, Padovani A, Scheltens P, et al. Timely diagnosis for Alzheimer's disease: a literature review on benefits and challenges. J Alzheimers Dis 2016; 49(3):617–31.

7. Jack CR Jr, Wiste HJ, Weigand SD, et al. Defining imaging biomarker cut points for brain aging and Alzheimer's disease. Alzheimers Dement 2017; 13(3):205–16.

8. Neale N, Padilla C, Fonseca LM, et al. Neuroimaging and other modalities to assess Alzheimer's disease in Down syndrome. Neuroimage Clin 2018;17: 263–71.

9. Stam CJ. Dementia and EEG. In: Lopes da Silva FH, Schomer DL, editors. Niedermeyer's electroencephalography: basic principles, clinical application and related fields. Lippincott Williams & Wilkins; 2012. p. 375–93.

10. Winblad B, Palmer K, Kivipelto M, et al. Mild cognitive impairment–beyond controversies, towards a consensus: report of the International Working Group on mild cognitive impairment. J Intern Med 2004;256(3):240–6.

11. Berger H. Uber das Elektrenkephalogramm des Menchen. Dritte Miteilung. Arch Psychiatr Nervenkr 1931;94:16–60.

12. Berger H. Uber das Elektrenkephalogramm des Menchen. Funfte Miteilung. Arch Psychiatr Nervenkr 1932;98:231–54.

13. Buchan RJ, Nagata K, Yokoyama E, et al. Regional correlations between the EEG and oxygen metabolism in dementia of Alzheimer's type. Electroencephalogr Clin Neurophysiol 1997;103(3):409–17.

14. Claus JJ, Ongerboer De Visser BW, Bour LJ, et al. Determinants of quantitative spectral electroencephalography in early Alzheimer's disease: cognitive function, regional cerebral blood flow, and computed tomography. Dement Geriatr Cogn Disord 2000;11(2):81–9.

15. Huang C, Wahlund L, Dierks T, et al. Discrimination of Alzheimer's disease and mild cognitive impairment by equivalent EEG sources: a cross-sectional and longitudinal study. Clin Neurophysiol 2000;111(11):1961–7.

16. Dierks T, Jelic V, Pascual-Marqui RD, et al. Spatial pattern of cerebral glucose metabolism (PET) correlates with localization of intracerebral EEG-generators in Alzheimer's disease. Clin Neurophysiol 2000;111(10):1817–24.

17. Chiang AKI, Rennie CJ, Robinson PA, et al. Age trends and sex differences of alpha rhythms including split alpha peaks. Clin Neurophysiol 2011;122(8):1505–17.

18. Samson-Dollfus D, Delapierre G, Do Marcolino C, et al. Normal and pathological changes in alpha rhythms. Int J Psychophysiol 1997;26(1–3):395–409.

19. Dierks T, Ihl R, Frölich L, et al. Dementia of the Alzheimer type: effects on the spontaneous EEG described by dipole sources. Psychiatry Res 1993; 50(3):151–62.

20. Riekkinen P, Buzsaki G, Riekkinen P Jr, et al. The cholinergic system and EEG slow waves. Electroencephalogr Clin Neurophysiol 1991;78(2):89–96.

21. Soininen H, Riekkinen P, Partanen VJ, et al. Alzheimer disease. In: Becker RE, Giacobini E, editors. Current research and early diagnosis. Taylor and Francis; 1990. p. 159–69.

22. Kikuchi M, Wada Y, Koshino Y, et al. Effects of scopolamine on interhemispheric EEG coherence in healthy subjects: analysis during rest and photic stimulation. Clin Electroencephalogr 2000;31(2): 109–15.

23. Dringenberg HC. Alzheimer's disease: more than a "cholinergic disorder" — evidence that cholinergic-monoaminergic interactions contribute to EEG slowing and dementia. Behav Brain Res 2000;115(2): 235–49.

24. Delbeuck X, Collette F, Van der Linden M. Is Alzheimer's disease a disconnection syndrome? Neuropsychologia 2007;45(14):3315–23.

25. Gloor P, Ball G, Schaul N. Brain lesions that produce delta waves in the EEG. Neurology 1977;27(4): 326–33.

26. Holschneider DP, Leuchter AF. Beta activity in aging and dementia. Brain Topogr 1995;8(2):169–80.

27. Saletu B, Anderer P, Paulus E, et al. EEG brain mapping in diagnostic and therapeutic assessment of dementia. Alzheimer Dis Assoc Disord 1991;5: S57–75.

28. Babiloni C, Frisoni GB, Pievani M, et al. Hippocampal volume and cortical sources of EEG alpha rhythms in mild cognitive impairment and Alzheimer disease. Neuroimage 2009;44(1):123–35.

29. Lehtovirta M, Partanen J, Könönen M, et al. A longitudinal quantitative EEG study of Alzheimer's disease: relation to apolipoprotein E polymorphism. Dement Geriatr Cogn Disord 2000; 11(1):29–35.

30. Lehtovirta M, Partanen J, Könönen M, et al. Spectral analysis of EEG in Alzheimer's disease: relation to apolipoprotein E polymorphism. Neurobiol Aging 1996;17(4):523–6.

31. Pekkonen E, Huotilainen M, Virtanen J, et al. Alzheimer's disease affects parallel processing between the auditory cortices. Neuroreport 1996;7(8):1365–8.

32. Pekkonen E, Jääskeläinen IP, Hietanen M, et al. Impaired preconscious auditory processing and cognitive functions in Alzheimer's disease. Clin Neurophysiol 1999;110(11):1942–7.

33. Berendse HW, Verbunt JP, Scheltens P, et al. Magnetoencephalographic analysis of cortical activity in Alzheimer's disease: a pilot study. Clin Neurophysiol 2000;111(4):604–12.

34. Fernández A, Hornero R, Mayo A, et al. Quantitative magnetoencephalography of spontaneous brain activity in Alzheimer disease: an exhaustive frequency analysis. Alzheimer Dis Assoc Disord 2006;20(3):153–9.

35. Fernández A, Hornero R, Mayo A, et al. MEG spectral profile in Alzheimer's disease and mild cognitive impairment. Clin Neurophysiol 2006;117(2):306–14.

36. López ME, Cuesta P, Garcés P, et al. MEG spectral analysis in subtypes of mild cognitive impairment. Age (Dordr) 2014;36(3):9624.

37. Fernández A, Maestú F, Amo C, et al. Focal temporoparietal slow activity in Alzheimer's disease revealed by magnetoencephalography. Biol Psychiatry 2002;52(7):764–70.

38. Fernández A, Arrazola J, Maestú F, et al. Correlations of hippocampal atrophy and focal low-frequency magnetic activity in Alzheimer disease: volumetric MR imaging-magnetoencephalographic study. AJNR Am J Neuroradiol 2003;24(3):481–7.

39. Osipova D, Ahveninen J, Jensen O, et al. Altered generation of spontaneous oscillations in Alzheimer's disease. Neuroimage 2005;27(4):835–41.

40. Osipova D, Rantanen K, Ahveninen J, et al. Source estimation of spontaneous MEG oscillations in mild cognitive impairment. Neurosci Lett 2006;405(1–2):57–61.

41. Engels MMA, Hillebrand A, van der Flier WM, et al. Slowing of hippocampal activity correlates with cognitive decline in early onset Alzheimer's disease. An MEG study with virtual electrodes. Front Hum Neurosci 2016;10:238.

42. López-Sanz D, Bruña R, Garcés P, et al. Alpha band disruption in the AD-continuum starts in the subjective cognitive decline stage: a MEG study. Sci Rep 2016;6:37685.

43. López-Sanz D, Bruña R, Garcés P, et al. Functional connectivity disruption in subjective cognitive decline and mild cognitive impairment: a common pattern of alterations. Front Aging Neurosci 2017;9:109.

44. López-Sanz D, Garcés P, Álvarez B, et al. Network Disruption in the Preclinical Stages of Alzheimer's Disease: From Subjective Cognitive Decline to Mild Cognitive Impairment. Int J Neural Syst 2017;27(8):1750041.

45. Garcia-Marin V, Blazquez-Llorca L, Rodriguez J-R, et al. Diminished perisomatic GABAergic terminals on cortical neurons adjacent to amyloid plaques. Front Neuroanat 2009;3:28.

46. Busche MA, Konnerth A. Impairments of neural circuit function in Alzheimer's disease. Philos Trans R Soc Lond B Biol Sci 2016;371(1700). https://doi.org/10.1098/rstb.2015.0429.

47. Sepulcre J, Sabuncu MR, Li Q, et al. Tau and amyloid β proteins distinctively associate to functional network changes in the aging brain. Alzheimers Dement 2017;13(11):1261–9.

48. Teipel SJ, Wohlert A, Metzger C, et al. Multicenter stability of resting state fMRI in the detection of Alzheimer's disease and amnestic MCI. Neuroimage Clin 2017;14:183–94.

49. Taniguchi T, Kawamata T, Mukai H, et al. Phosphorylation of tau is regulated by PKN. J Biol Chem 2001;276(13):10025–31.

50. Albert M, Zhu Y, Moghekar A, et al. Predicting progression from normal cognition to mild cognitive impairment for individuals at 5 years. Brain 2018;141(3):877–87.

51. Schultz AP, Chhatwal JP, Hedden T, et al. Phases of hyperconnectivity and hypoconnectivity in the default mode and salience networks track with amyloid and tau in clinically normal individuals. J Neurosci 2017;37(16):4323–31.

52. Delbeuck X, Van der Linden M, Collette F. Alzheimer's disease as a disconnection syndrome? Neuropsychol Rev 2003;13(2):79–92.

53. Selkoe DJ. Alzheimer's disease is a synaptic failure. Science 2002;298(5594):789–91.

54. Maestú F, Campo P, Del Río D, et al. Increased biomagnetic activity in the ventral pathway in mild cognitive impairment. Clin Neurophysiol 2008;119(6):1320–7.

55. Stam CJ, de Haan W, Daffertshofer A, et al. Graph theoretical analysis of magnetoencephalographic functional connectivity in Alzheimer's disease. Brain 2009;132(Pt 1):213–24.

56. Buldú JM, Bajo R, Maestú F, et al. Reorganization of functional networks in mild cognitive impairment. PLoS One 2011;6(5):e19584.

57. Maestú F, Peña J-M, Garcés P, et al. A multicenter study of the early detection of synaptic dysfunction in mild cognitive impairment using magnetoencephalography-derived functional connectivity. Neuroimage Clin 2015;9:103–9.

58. López ME, Bruña R, Aurtenetxe S, et al. Alpha-band hypersynchronization in progressive mild cognitive

impairment: a magnetoencephalography study. J Neurosci 2014;34(44):14551–9.

59. Bajo R, Maestú F, Nevado A, et al. Functional connectivity in mild cognitive impairment during a memory task: implications for the disconnection hypothesis. J Alzheimers Dis 2010;22(1): 183–93.

60. Fernández A, Turrero A, Zuluaga P, et al. Magnetoencephalographic parietal δ dipole density in mild cognitive impairment: preliminary results of a method to estimate the risk of developing Alzheimer disease. Arch Neurol 2006;63(3):427–30.

61. Fernández A, Turrero A, Zuluaga P, et al. MEG delta mapping along the healthy aging-Alzheimer's disease continuum: diagnostic implications. J Alzheimers Dis 2013;35(3):495–507.

62. López ME, Turrero A, Cuesta P, et al. Searching for primary predictors of conversion from mild cognitive impairment to Alzheimer's disease: a multivariate follow-up study. J Alzheimers Dis 2016;52(1): 133–43.

63. Bajo R, Castellanos NP, Cuesta P, et al. Differential patterns of connectivity in progressive mild cognitive impairment. Brain Connect 2012;2(1):21–4.

64. Canuet L, Pusil S, López ME, et al. Network disruption and cerebrospinal fluid amyloid-beta and phospho-tau levels in mild cognitive impairment. J Neurosci 2015;35(28):10325–30.

65. Nakamura A, Cuesta P, Kato T, et al. Early functional network alterations in asymptomatic elders at risk for Alzheimer's disease. Sci Rep 2017;7(1):6517.

66. Nakamura A, Cuesta P, Fernández A, et al. Electromagnetic signatures of the preclinical and prodromal stages of Alzheimer's disease. Brain 2018; 141(5):1470–85.

67. Braak H, Braak E. Neuropathological staging of Alzheimer-related changes. Acta Neuropathol 1991; 82(4):239–59.

68. Fornito A, Zalesky A, Breakspear M. The connectomics of brain disorders. Nat Rev Neurosci 2015; 16(3):159–72.

69. Cuesta P, Garcés P, Castellanos NP, et al. Influence of the APOE ε4 allele and mild cognitive impairment diagnosis in the disruption of the MEG resting state functional connectivity in sources space. J Alzheimers Dis 2015;44(2): 493–505.

70. Cuesta P, Barabash A, Aurtenetxe S, et al. Source analysis of spontaneous magnetoencephalograpic activity in healthy aging and mild cognitive impairment: influence of apolipoprotein E polymorphism. J Alzheimers Dis 2015;43(1): 259–73.

71. Garcés P, Martín-Buro MC, Maestú F. Quantifying the test-retest reliability of magnetoencephalography resting-state functional connectivity. Brain Connect 2016;6(6):448–60.

Magnetoencephalography and Language

Suzanne Dikker, PhD[a],*, M. Florencia Assaneo, PhD[a], Laura Gwilliams, MSc[a,b], Lin Wang, PhD[c], Anne Kösem, PhD[d]

KEYWORDS

• MEG • Language • Speech • Reading • Neurolinguistics • Synchronization • Decoding • Semantics

KEY POINTS

- Its high temporal resolution and relatively accurate spatial resolution make magnetoencephalography (MEG) an ideal tool to investigate the complex brain dynamics supporting language comprehension and production.
- Event-related designs using single words or simple, well-controlled phrases have helped characterize the building blocks of language as well as the different linguistic processing stages, from identifying sounds to syntactic phrase building.
- More recent methodological approaches, such as investigating neural oscillations and decoding techniques, allow researchers to study dynamic naturalistic language comprehension and production.
- Linguistically relevant brain MEG responses are atypical in language disorders.

INTRODUCTION

Language is among the most complex of human cognitive systems, yet its processing is extremely automated and fast: Both behavioral and neurophysiological studies suggest that within 600 ms of a word's onset, its sensory properties have been analyzed, its grammatical and semantic features have been retrieved from memory, and it has been integrated into the ongoing discourse. In this article, we provide a brief overview, summarized in **Fig. 1**, of research that has capitalized on the spatio-temporal resolution of magnetoencephalography (MEG) to capture the neural dynamics that support linguistic operations. First, we review event-related designs using single words or simple, well-controlled phrases, which have helped characterize the building blocks of language and its processing stages, from identifying individual sounds or letters to sentence-level grammar. We then discuss more recent methodological approaches exploring neural oscillations and decoding techniques, which can be applied to naturalistic language. These tools have allowed researchers to study how linguistically relevant brain responses are coupled between brain regions and across modalities, and to capture language-relevant brain responses that are highly distributed across space and vary in timing. We conclude with a brief section exemplifying the clinical relevance of the reviewed research.

EVOKED RESPONSES TO LINGUISTIC INPUT
Early Brain Responses to Written Words

In a now classic study, Tarkiainen and colleagues[1] compared brain responses to symbols and letter strings and identified 2 early event-related MEG

a Department of Psychology, New York University, 6 Washington Place #275, New York, NY 10003, USA; b New York University Abu Dhabi Research Institute, New York University Abu Dhabi, Saadiyat Island, Abu Dhabi, United Arab Emirates; c Department of Psychiatry, Athinoula A. Martinos Center for Biomedical Imaging, Massachusetts General Hospital, Harvard Medical School, 149 Thirteenth Street, #2306, Charlestown, MA 02129, USA; d Lyon Neuroscience Research Center (CRNL), CH Le Vinatier Bâtiment 452, 95, BD Pinel, Bron, Lyon 69675, France
* Corresponding author.
E-mail address: suzanne.dikker@nyu.edu

Neuroimag Clin N Am 30 (2020) 229–238
https://doi.org/10.1016/j.nic.2020.01.004

responses to visual word recognition.[1] Later studies have built on this work to identify early language-related MEG components, or event-related fields (ERFs).[2,3] As listed in **Fig. 1**, the so-called visual M100 response has been associated with low-level visual feature processing,[4] the M130 component shows sensitivity to orthographic features[3] (e.g., how often 2 letters co-occur in written words), and the M170 response is sensitive to the morphologic properties of words.[5] For a review see Gwilliams (2020).[6] For example, bimorphemic words elicit a higher M170 amplitude than orthographically matched monomorphemic words ("farm-er" has 2

morphemes, or meaningful units, vs "corner," which consists of 1 morpheme but also ends in "-er"[5]). Functional magnetic resonance imaging (fMRI) evidence from manipulations similar to those affecting the M170 suggests that the response is generated in left and right fusiform gyri.[7]

Identifying Phonetic and Morphemic Information in Spoken Language

Systematic early responses to *spoken* language also can be identified. Relative to the onset of each speech sound, evoked responses at 50 ms

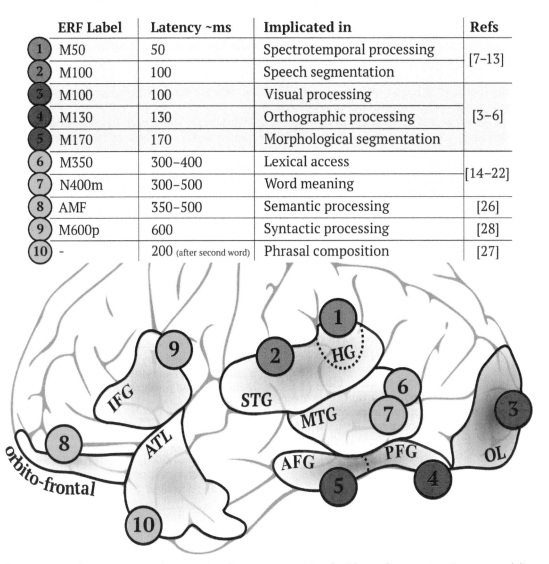

	ERF Label	Latency ~ms	Implicated in	Refs
1	M50	50	Spectrotemporal processing	[7–13]
2	M100	100	Speech segmentation	
3	M100	100	Visual processing	
4	M130	130	Orthographic processing	[3–6]
5	M170	170	Morphological segmentation	
6	M350	300–400	Lexical access	[14–22]
7	N400m	300–500	Word meaning	
8	AMF	350–500	Semantic processing	[26]
9	M600p	600	Syntactic processing	[28]
10	-	200 (after second word)	Phrasal composition	[27]

Fig. 1. Putative brain regions and event-related responses associated with word processing. Orange: modality-specific written word processes. Purple: modality-specific spoken word processes. Turquoise: a-modal processes. AFG, anterior fusiform gyrus; ATL, anterior temporal lobe; HG, Heschl gyrus; IFG, inferior frontal gyrus; MTG, middle temporal gyrus; OL, occipital lobe; PFG, posterior fusiform gyrus; STG, superior temporal gyrus. (*Adapted from* Gwilliams L. How the brain composes morphemes into meaning. Phil Trans R Soc B 2020;375(1791):20190311; with permission.)

in primary auditory cortex are modulated by low-level spectro-temporal properties of the input, followed by a 100 ms response in superior temporal gyrus.[8–11] This latter response has been associated with the mapping of variable acoustic information onto more stable phonetic features (eg, the acoustics of [p] vary between speakers and contexts, like in [plant] vs [park], but these different sounds are mapped onto a single meaningful phoneme in the perceiver's brain).[12]

Having identified the phonemes, these are then mapped onto words (via morphemes, see earlier in this article). This process has been explained through the prevalent *cohort model* of spoken word recognition (Fig. 2): as a listener hears each phoneme of a word (i.e., the spoken equivalent of a letter), this information is used to narrow down the cohort of words that are consistent with the input. When just 1 word remains, this is the winner of the lexical competition, and thus the word that is recognized. Previous MEG studies have found evidence in favor of this mechanism by tracking responses to each speech sound in the word, and correlating activity at approximately 200 ms after phoneme onset in the superior temporal gyrus with the number of remaining morphologic candidates[11,13,14] (see Fig. 2).

Deriving the Meaning of Words in Isolation and in Context

Once the words have been identified, their meaning can be derived. A large body of MEG studies have compared evoked brain responses to words differing in lexical properties (words vs nonwords; abstract vs concrete words[2]), preceding word contexts (eg, "dog" followed by "cat" vs "dog" followed by "table"[15,16]), or sentence contexts (eg, "mountain" vs "tulip" in "The climbers finally reached the top of the ..."[17–19]; Fig. 3A). When semantic features of a word are easier to access, smaller evoked MEG responses are observed approximately 300 to 500 ms after word onset (corresponding to the N400 in an electroencephalogram [EEG][20]). This N400m effect has been consistently localized within the left lateral temporal cortex, including superior and middle temporal regions (Fig. 3B).

This is in line with the well-established role of these regions in representing lexico-semantic information, as revealed by fMRI.[21] Importantly, although early ERFs are modality specific, semantic activation appears to be modality-independent: overlapping brain regions are activated during the N400m time window for both written and spoken language.[22] In addition to the left temporal cortex, a number of MEG studies report increased activation within the left inferior frontal cortex for semantically incongruous words.[23,24] This region has been suggested to play a role in selecting and controlling lexical retrieval under contextual influence[17,25] and in unifying multiple sources of information.[26]

Combining Words: Syntax and Sentence-Level Semantics

Although the bulk of studies focus on processing word meaning, research has also examined

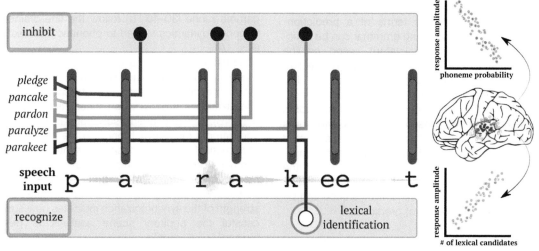

Fig. 2. Schematic of spoken word recognition. As the word unfolds, with each phoneme (*gray bars*), possible lexical candidates for recognition are ruled out. This process continues until only one word remains consistent with the input (e.g., "parakeet"). Notice that the word can be uniquely identified before word offset: at the "k" phoneme. Activity in the left superior temporal gyrus has been shown to track the probability of each phoneme in a word ("phoneme surprisal"), as well as the relative probability of remaining lexical candidates ("cohort entropy").

A Sensor-level evoked response

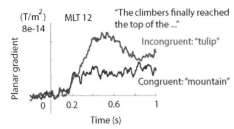

B Source localization of the evoked response difference

left superior temporal gyrus: incongruent > congruent

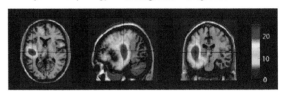

Fig. 3. Evoked responses to words in expected vs unexpected contexts. (*A*) The planar gradient of the ERFs time-locked to the onset of the critical words at a representative left temporal sensor. Between approximately 200 ms and 700 ms after the critical words, the incongruent words (e.g., "tulip") elicited larger amplitudes than the congruent words (e.g., "mountain"). (*B*) Source localization of the N400m effect using minimum-norm estimate. MLT, middle temporal lobe. (*Adapted from* L Wang, O Jensen, D van den Brink, et al. Beta oscillations relate to the N400m during language comprehension. Human Brain Mapp, 2012 33(12), 2898–2912; with permission.)

sentence-level combinatorics.[27,28] For example, when comparing the word "boat" in either a word list or as part of the phrase "red boat", the latter leads to linguistic composition-related activity in the left anterior temporal lobe and ventromedial prefrontal cortex (e.g.,[29] see **Fig. 1**). Also, "going" vs "go" in a sentence like "She will *going/go* to the bakery for a loaf of bread"[30] elicit a stronger response after 600 ms, consistently source-localized to temporal regions, corresponding to the P600 effect observed in EEG research.[31]

Syntactically incongruous words sometimes also elicit stronger early *sensory* responses than grammatical sentences, as early as 100 ms after word onset.[4,32–34] Recall that research investigating words in isolation yielded no evidence that the brain is sensitive to lexical or grammatical properties in sensory cortices. This discrepancy between word-level and sentence-level findings has been explained in terms of a prediction-based account: words and grammar can be anticipated (and thus preactivated) based on the preceding context, allowing for a more efficient detection of linguistically relevant features. For example, the brain may generate estimates about the likely physical appearance of upcoming words based on grammar-based predictions, and words that do not "look" or "sound" like the expected grammatical category then show increased amplitude in early sensory responses. Many of the studies cited previously in relation to lexical-semantic processing have similarly accounted for N400m effects in terms of prediction.[15,35,36]

BEYOND EVENT-RELATED FIELDS AND TOWARD NATURALISTIC EXPERIMENTATION

In recent years, a shift has been made toward a more naturalistic experimental setup (eg, Ref.[37]) in which participants listen to continuous speech,

such as stories, rather than being presented with isolated words or short sentences. As the evoked response to natural language at a certain time point may reflect a cascade of processes initiated at different (and overlapping) moments in time, researchers have resorted to other analysis techniques to study continuous speech.

The Role of Neural Oscillations in Language

Tracking continuous speech: brain-to-stimulus synchrony

There is strong evidence that brain oscillations synchronize to the temporal regularities of speech during listening[38–41]: low-frequency neural oscillations in the theta and delta range (1–8 Hz) synchronize to the dynamics of the speech envelope associated with syllabic and phrasal rates respectively, and high-frequency neural activity in the gamma range (30–40 Hz) follow the fine-grained temporal dynamics related to phonetic features[42] (**Fig. 4**A).

Neural oscillations have been experimentally linked to understanding speech (i.e., beyond mere speech acoustics): brain-to-speech synchronization is stronger when speech is intelligible (**Fig. 4**B),[43–45] and brain oscillations in the delta and gamma range synchronize to the lexical and grammatical structures of spoken sentences.[46–48] In multitalker settings, neural oscillations synchronize to the dynamics of the attended speaker (the so-called "cocktail party effect"). Importantly, the strength of the synchronization indicates how successful the auditory scene analysis is performed[49–51] (**Fig. 4**C).

Neural oscillations are hypothesized to play a crucial role during speech parsing by defining the temporal boundaries between linguistic items within the continuous acoustic signal.[42] Importantly, brain-to-speech synchrony is suggested

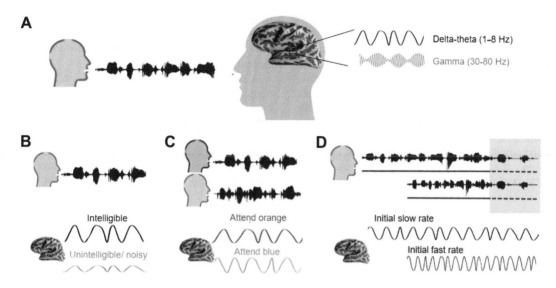

Fig. 4. Brain-to-stimulus synchrony and speech processing. (*A*) Brain signal synchronizes to the dynamics of speech. (*B*) Brain-to-stimulus synchrony is stronger when speech is intelligible.[43–45] (*C*) Brain oscillations follow attended speech in multitalker settings.[49–51] (*D*) Brain oscillations are influenced by contextual speech rhythm information.[54] (*Courtesy of* A Kösem, PhD, Boulevard Pinel, Bron, France.)

to be a predictive mechanism, parsing and structuring events from continuous speech by building temporal expectations on the upcoming auditory input.[52,53] In support of this view, neural oscillations entrain to the syllabic rate of speech in a sustained manner, and neural entrainment to ongoing speech is dependent on the rate of preceding speech. Importantly, brain-to-speech synchrony at specific rates directly affects how words are understood[54] (**Fig. 4**D).

The role of neural oscillations in deriving meaning

Examining oscillatory activity has also allowed researchers to closely track the cortical dynamics underlying semantic processing in event-related designs, substantially enriching the information obtained by studying ERFs. For example, during sentence comprehension, desynchronization of neural oscillations in the alpha (8–12 Hz) and beta (12–20 Hz) ranges within the left temporal and frontal regions is observed when processing semantically anomalous (vs congruent) words in sentence contexts[19,30,55] or for words appearing in sentences vs word lists.[56] The desynchronized alpha/beta activity might reflect the engagement of task-relevant brain regions to support sentence-level processing. Furthermore, connectivity analyses in MEG studies have revealed functional connectivity patterns between the left inferior frontal and temporal cortex during sentence comprehension. Granger causality analysis

suggests that alpha activity supports information transfer from temporal to frontal regions, whereas beta activity supports information transfer from frontal to temporal regions.[57] The connectivity between the left frontal and temporal regions was also found by synchronized beta and low-gamma oscillations for processing unexpected compared with expected sentence-final words.[58] Moreover, cross-frequency connectivity between gamma power within the left prefrontal region and alpha power within the left temporal region was reported for processing expected but not unexpected sentence-final words, both before and after the words were presented.[55] These findings suggest that the communication between the left inferior frontal and temporal cortex is supported by different patterns of oscillatory activity. Further studies are needed to systematically examine how the communication between different brain regions (e.g., feedforward vs feedback control) is realized via different patterns of synchronization (e.g., phase-locking, amplitude synchronization, phase-amplitude coupling) in different frequency bands.[55,59]

Auditory-motor interaction in speech

In the middle of the 20th century, researchers observed that phonemes cannot be unequivocally defined in the acoustic space, and proposed that phoneme perception instead occurs in motor space: incoming speech sounds are mapped to invariant neuromotor commands.[60,61] This hypothesis, dubbed the *motor theory of speech perception*, has been strongly criticized,[62–67] but less stringent versions are supported by findings that passive listening to speech activates areas involved in speech production.[68,69] MEG data show that oscillations generated in left inferior frontal and precentral gyri (areas typically involved in speech production) modulate the phase of low-frequency activity in left auditory regions significantly stronger when speech is intelligible than when it is unintelligible (e.g., backward speech). This top-down control leads

to a better tracking of the speech envelope by the auditory cortex activity,[70,71] suggesting that motor areas help enhance auditory temporal prediction during speech processing.[52]

In recent MEG research in which participants passively listened to rhythmic strings of syllables,[72] the synchronization between auditory and motor regions was found to be highest when syllables were presented at a rate of 4.5 syllables per second (**Fig. 5**), corresponding to the mean syllable rate of natural speech across languages.[73] One plausible explanation is that speech

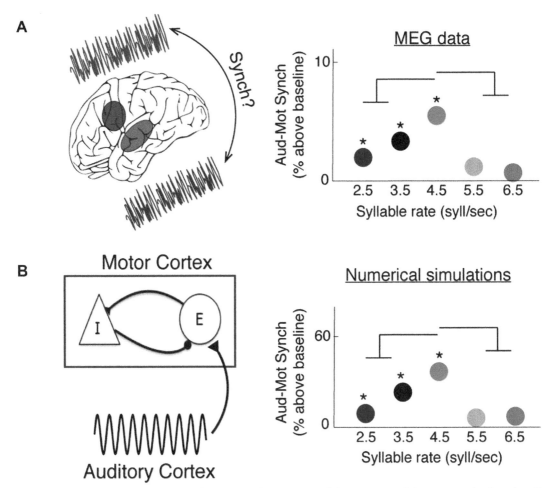

Fig. 5. Auditory-motor synchronization during speech perception. (*A*) Experimental data. Motor (*red*) and auditory (*blue*) cortical activity was recorded while participants passively listened to rhythmic train of syllables at different rates. The synchronization between cortices significantly increased from baseline just if syllables were presented at 2.5, 3.5, and 4.5 syllables per second (syll/s) and was enhanced at the central condition (4.5 syll/s). (*B*) Model output. Motor cortex (*red box*) was modeled through a set of Wilson-Cowan equations representing an inhibitory-excitatory network, and the excitatory population receives the auditory cortex activity (*blue signal*) as input. The Wilson-Cowan is a biophysically inspired model, which behaves as a neural oscillator. Numerical simulation obtained by setting the natural frequency of the oscillator at 4.5 Hz reproduced the experimental pattern of auditory-motor synchrony. Asterisks stand for significant differences (*P*<.05). (*Adapted from* MF Assaneo, D Poeppel. The coupling between auditory and motor cortices is rate-restricted: Evidence for an intrinsic speech-motor rhythm. Science Advances. 2018;4(2); with permission.)

production regions behave as a neural oscillator (a system capable of generating oscillations at its own natural frequency and showing entrainment to a rhythmic stimulus only if the external frequency is close to its natural one[74]) with a natural frequency close to 4.5 Hz. Thus, the temporal patterns of speech could emerge as a consequence of the intrinsic rhythms of cortical areas.

Decoding Approaches in Language Research

Another approach that has gained popularity in recent years is "multivariate" or "decoding" analyses. For MEG, this typically involves using the activity pattern across all sensors (not just one location at a time; hence, "multi-" variate) to read out the stimulus property as it is encoded in the neural response (hence, "decoding"). The algorithms for this approach have been largely borrowed from the machine-learning community, and can provide an increased sensitivity in situations in which the neural processes do not necessarily evoke a strong focal amplitude modulation. For example, evidence from a decoding analysis on EEG-MEG data, aimed at differentiating responses to words of different semantic categories (e.g., living vs nonliving), suggests that relevant responses are not only highly distributed across space, but also vary in temporal pattern.[75] Further, a recent study demonstrated the ability to decode the identity of a word before it begins, when that word is highly predictable in context.[55] This was achieved by examining the spatial pattern of brain activity before the presentation of predicted words. Overall, these studies show that applying multivariate analysis to the MEG data paves the way for studying language processing in cases in which classic evoked-response analysis would not be sensitive to the true underlying processing differences.

CLINICAL RELEVANCE

Disrupted evoked responses to speech and text have been associated with several language deficits. For example, dyslexic participants exhibit atypical early evoked responses to letters,[76] and N400m responses measured in infancy can predict reading speed in adolescence for children at risk for dyslexia.[77] Disruption of early neural processing to speech sounds has also been linked to dyslexia, as well as specific language impairment (SLI).[78,79]

The study of neural oscillations and their link to speech and language disorders is also receiving increasing interest. Hearing impairment affects alpha oscillations and speech-brain synchronization; both oscillatory deficits are associated with the degree of hearing loss in noisy environments.[80] Dyslexia and SLI have been proposed to originate from abnormal neural oscillatory profiles in response to speech[81,82]: children who have inefficient brain-to-speech synchronization may have a harder time segmenting the acoustic signal, leading to language difficulties.[83,84] Individuals with dyslexia show stronger synchronization to fast auditory rhythms in the gamma range (40 Hz) as compared with controls, suggesting disrupted auditory timing processing for phoneme perception.[85] Brain synchronization to the slower dynamics of the speech envelope is also disrupted in dyslexia and SLI.[86–88]

To remediate language deficits, rhythm training programs have been tested to improve speech timing perception based on finger-tapping or musical exposure.[89,90] Finger-tapping and musical exposure have both been associated with increased recruitment of neural oscillations.[91,92] Ongoing research is currently investigating the direct link between neural oscillatory activity and speech perception improvement during training.

ACKNOWLEDGMENTS

This work is supported by NIH 2R01DC05660, NSF ECR-1661016, Marie Sklodowska-Curie Individual Fellowship MSCA-IF-2018-843088, and Abu Dhabi Institute Grant G1001.

DISCLOSURE

All authors report that they have no conflict of interest.

REFERENCES

1. Tarkiainen A, Helenius P, Hansen PC, et al. Dynamics of letter string perception in the human occipitotemporal cortex. Brain 1999;122(Pt 11):2119–32.
2. Pylkkänen L, Marantz A. Tracking the time course of word recognition with MEG. Trends Cogn Sci 2003; 7(5):187–9.
3. Gwilliams L, Lewis GA, Marantz A. Functional characterisation of letter-specific responses in time, space and current polarity using magnetoencephalography. Neuroimage 2016;132:320–33.
4. Dikker S, Rabagliati H, Pylkkänen L. Sensitivity to syntax in visual cortex. Cognition 2009;110(3): 293–321.
5. Zweig E, Pylkkänen L. A visual M170 effect of morphological complexity. Lang Cogn Process 2009;24(3):412–39.
6. Gwilliams L. How the brain composes morphemes into meaning. Phil Trans R Soc B 2020;375(1791): 20190311.

7. McCandliss BD, Cohen L, Dehaene S. The visual word form area: expertise for reading in the fusiform gyrus. Trends Cogn Sci 2003;7(7):293–9.

8. Chang EF, Rieger JW, Johnson K, et al. Categorical speech representation in human superior temporal gyrus. Nat Neurosci 2010;13(11):1428–32.

9. Mesgarani N, Cheung C, Johnson K, et al. Phonetic feature encoding in human superior temporal gyrus. Science 2014;343(6174):1006–10.

10. Di Liberto GM, O'Sullivan JA, Lalor EC. Low-frequency cortical entrainment to speech reflects phoneme-level processing. Curr Biol 2015;25(19): 2457–65.

11. Gwilliams L, Poeppel D, Marantz A, et al. Phonological (un)certainty weights lexical activation. Proceedings of the 8th Workshop on Cognitive Modeling and Computational Linguistics (CMCL 2018). 2018. doi:10.18653/v1/w18-0104

12. Gwilliams L, Linzen T, Poeppel D, et al. In spoken word recognition, the future predicts the past. J Neurosci 2018;38(35):7585–99.

13. Ettinger A, Linzen T, Marantz A. The role of morphology in phoneme prediction: evidence from MEG. Brain Lang 2014;129:14–23.

14. Gwilliams L, Marantz A. Non-linear processing of a linear speech stream: the influence of morphological structure on the recognition of spoken Arabic words. Brain Lang 2015;147:1–13.

15. Lau EF, Weber K, Gramfort A, et al. Spatiotemporal signatures of lexical–semantic prediction. Cereb Cortex 2016;26(4):1377–87.

16. Vistoli D, Passerieux C, Houze B, et al. Neural basis of semantic priming in schizophrenia during a lexical decision task: a magneto-encephalography study. Schizophr Res 2011;130(1–3):114–22.

17. Lau EF, Phillips C, Poeppel D. A cortical network for semantics: (de)constructing the N400. Nat Rev Neurosci 2008;9(12):920–33.

18. Maess B, Herrmann CS, Hahne A, et al. Localizing the distributed language network responsible for the N400 measured by MEG during auditory sentence processing. Brain Res 2006;1096(1): 163–72.

19. Wang L, Jensen O, van den Brink D, et al. Beta oscillations relate to the N400m during language comprehension. Hum Brain Mapp 2012;33(12): 2898–912.

20. Kutas M, Federmeier KD. Thirty years and counting: finding meaning in the N400 component of the event-related brain potential (ERP). Annu Rev Psychol 2011;62:621–47.

21. Binder JR, Desai RH, Graves WW, et al. Where is the semantic system? A critical review and meta-analysis of 120 functional neuroimaging studies. Cereb Cortex 2009;19(12):2767–96.

22. Marinkovic K, Dhond RP, Dale AM, et al. Spatiotemporal dynamics of modality-specific and supramodal word processing. Neuron 2003;38(3): 487–97.

23. Halgren E, Dhond RP, Christensen N, et al. N400-like magnetoencephalography responses modulated by semantic context, word frequency, and lexical class in sentences. Neuroimage 2002;17(3):1101–16.

24. Pylkkänen L, Oliveri B, Smart AJ. Semantics vs. world knowledge in prefrontal cortex. Lang Cogn Process 2009;24(9):1313–34.

25. Bedny M, McGill M, Thompson-Schill SL. Semantic adaptation and competition during word comprehension. Cereb Cortex 2008;18(11):2574–85.

26. Hagoort P, Indefrey P. The neurobiology of language beyond single words. Annu Rev Neurosci 2014;37: 347–62.

27. Pylkkänen L, Martin AE, McElree B, et al. The anterior midline field: coercion or decision making? Brain Lang 2009;108(3):184–90.

28. Pylkkänen L. The neural basis of combinatory syntax and semantics. Science 2019;366(6461):62–6.

29. Bemis DK, Pylkkänen L. Simple composition: a magnetoencephalography investigation into the comprehension of minimal linguistic phrases. J Neurosci 2011;31(8):2801–14.

30. Kielar A, Panamsky L, Links KA, et al. Localization of electrophysiological responses to semantic and syntactic anomalies in language comprehension with MEG. Neuroimage 2015;105:507–24.

31. Osterhout L, Holcomb PJ. Event-related brain potentials elicited by syntactic anomaly. J Mem Lang 1992;31(6):785–806.

32. Dikker S, Rabagliati H, Farmer TA, et al. Early occipital sensitivity to syntactic category is based on form typicality. Psychol Sci 2010;21(5):629–34.

33. Herrmann B, Maess B, Hasting AS, et al. Localization of the syntactic mismatch negativity in the temporal cortex: an MEG study. Neuroimage 2009; 48(3):590–600.

34. Nieuwland MS. Do "early" brain responses reveal word form prediction during language comprehension? A critical review. Neurosci Biobehav Rev 2019;96:367–400.

35. Maess B, Mamashli F, Obleser J, et al. Prediction signatures in the brain: semantic pre-activation during language comprehension. Front Hum Neurosci 2016;10. https://doi.org/10.3389/fnhum.2016.00591.

36. Lau EF, Holcomb PJ, Kuperberg GR. Dissociating N400 effects of prediction from association in single-word contexts. J Cogn Neurosci 2013;25(3): 484–502.

37. Brennan J, Nir Y, Hasson U, et al. Syntactic structure building in the anterior temporal lobe during natural story listening. Brain Lang 2012;120(2):163–73.

38. Ahissar E, Nagarajan S, Ahissar M, et al. Speech comprehension is correlated with temporal response patterns recorded from auditory cortex. Proc Natl Acad Sci U S A 2001;98(23):13367–72.

39. Howard MF, Poeppel D. Discrimination of speech stimuli based on neuronal response phase patterns depends on acoustics but not comprehension. J Neurophysiol 2010;104(5):2500–11.

40. Luo H, Poeppel D. Phase patterns of neuronal responses reliably discriminate speech in human auditory cortex. Neuron 2007;54(6):1001–10.

41. Curio G, Neuloh G, Numminen J, et al. Speaking modifies voice-evoked activity in the human auditory cortex. Hum Brain Mapp 2000;9(4):183–91.

42. Giraud A-L, Poeppel D. Cortical oscillations and speech processing: emerging computational principles and operations. Nat Neurosci 2012;15(4):511–7.

43. Doelling KB, Arnal LH, Ghitza O, et al. Acoustic landmarks drive delta-theta oscillations to enable speech comprehension by facilitating perceptual parsing. Neuroimage 2014;85(Pt 2):761–8.

44. Peelle JE, Gross J, Davis MH. Phase-locked responses to speech in human auditory cortex are enhanced during comprehension. Cereb Cortex 2013;23(6):1378–87.

45. Ding N, Simon JZ. Adaptive temporal encoding leads to a background-insensitive cortical representation of speech. J Neurosci 2013;33(13):5728–35.

46. Ding N, Melloni L, Zhang H, et al. Cortical tracking of hierarchical linguistic structures in connected speech. Nat Neurosci 2016;19(1):158–64.

47. Kösem A, Basirat A, Azizi L, et al. High-frequency neural activity predicts word parsing in ambiguous speech streams. J Neurophysiol 2016;116(6):2497–512.

48. Meyer L, Henry MJ, Gaston P, et al. Linguistic bias modulates interpretation of speech via neural delta-band oscillations. Cereb Cortex 2017;27(9):4293–302.

49. Zion Golumbic EM, Ding N, Bickel S, et al. Mechanisms underlying selective neuronal tracking of attended speech at a "Cocktail Party". Neuron 2013;77(5):980–91.

50. Rimmele JM, Zion Golumbic E, Schröger E, et al. The effects of selective attention and speech acoustics on neural speech-tracking in a multi-talker scene. Cortex 2015;68:144–54.

51. Riecke L, Formisano E, Sorger B, et al. Neural entrainment to speech modulates speech intelligibility. Curr Biol 2018;28(2):161–9.e5.

52. Rimmele JM, Morillon B, Poeppel D, et al. Proactive sensing of periodic and aperiodic auditory patterns. Trends Cogn Sci 2018;22(10):870–82.

53. Morillon B, Schroeder CE. Neuronal oscillations as a mechanistic substrate of auditory temporal prediction. Ann N Y Acad Sci 2015;1337:26–31.

54. Kösem A, Bosker HR, Takashima A, et al. Neural entrainment determines the words we hear. Curr Biol 2018;28(18):2867–75.e3.

55. Wang L, Hagoort P, Jensen O. Language prediction is reflected by coupling between frontal gamma and posterior alpha oscillations. J Cogn Neurosci 2018; 30(3):432–47.

56. Lam NHL, Schoffelen J-M, Uddén J, et al. Neural activity during sentence processing as reflected in theta, alpha, beta, and gamma oscillations. Neuroimage 2016;142:43–54.

57. Schoffelen J-M, Hultén A, Lam N, et al. Frequency-specific directed interactions in the human brain network for language. Proc Natl Acad Sci U S A 2017;114(30):8083–8.

58. Mamashli F, Khan S, Obleser J, et al. Oscillatory dynamics of cortical functional connections in semantic prediction. Hum Brain Mapp 2019;40(6):1856–66.

59. Keitel A, Ince RAA, Gross J, et al. Auditory cortical delta-entrainment interacts with oscillatory power in multiple fronto-parietal networks. Neuroimage 2017;147:32–42.

60. Liberman AM, Cooper FS, Shankweiler DP, et al. Perception of the speech code. Psychol Rev 1967;74(6):431–61.

61. Liberman AM, Mattingly IG. The motor theory of speech perception revised. Cognition 1985;21(1):1–36.

62. Lane H. The motor theory of speech perception: a critical review. Psychol Rev 1965;72:275–309.

63. Massaro DW, Chen TH. The motor theory of speech perception revisited. Psychon Bull Rev 2008;15(2):453–7 [discussion: 458–62].

64. Galantucci B, Fowler CA, Turvey MT. The motor theory of speech perception reviewed. Psychon Bull Rev 2006;13(3):361–77.

65. Pulvermüller F, Fadiga L. Active perception: sensorimotor circuits as a cortical basis for language. Nat Rev Neurosci 2010;11(5):351–60.

66. Lotto AJ, Hickok GS, Holt LL. Reflections on mirror neurons and speech perception. Trends Cogn Sci 2009;13(3):110–4.

67. Skipper JI, Devlin JT, Lametti DR. The hearing ear is always found close to the speaking tongue: review of the role of the motor system in speech perception. Brain Lang 2017;164:77–105.

68. Wilson SM, Saygin AP, Sereno MI, et al. Listening to speech activates motor areas involved in speech production. Nat Neurosci 2004;7(7):701–2.

69. Pulvermüller F, Huss M, Kherif F, et al. Motor cortex maps articulatory features of speech sounds. Proc Natl Acad Sci U S A 2006;103(20):7865–70.

70. Park H, Ince RAA, Schyns PG, et al. Frontal top-down signals increase coupling of auditory low-frequency oscillations to continuous speech in human listeners. Curr Biol 2015;25(12):1649–53.

71. Park H, Thut G, Gross J. Predictive entrainment of natural speech through two fronto-motor top- down channels. Lang Cogn Neurosci 2018;1–13. https://doi.org/10.1080/23273798.2018.1506589.

72. Assaneo MF, Poeppel D. The coupling between auditory and motor cortices is rate-restricted: evidence for an intrinsic speech-motor rhythm. Sci Adv 2018;4(2):eaao3842.

73. Ding N, Patel AD, Chen L, et al. Temporal modulations in speech and music. Neurosci Biobehav Rev 2017;81(Pt B):181–7.

74. Hoppensteadt, Frank C, Eugene M. Izhikevich. Weakly connected neural networks. Springer Science & Business Media; 2012.

75. Chan AM, Halgren E, Marinkovic K, et al. Decoding word and category-specific spatiotemporal representations from MEG and EEG. Neuroimage 2011; 54(4):3028–39.

76. Helenius P, Tarkiainen A, Cornelissen P, et al. Dissociation of normal feature analysis and deficient processing of letter-strings in dyslexic adults. Cereb Cortex 1999;9(5):476–83.

77. Lohvansuu K, Hämäläinen JA, Ervast L, et al. Longitudinal interactions between brain and cognitive measures on reading development from 6 months to 14 years. Neuropsychologia 2018; 108:6–12.

78. Helenius P, Parviainen T, Paetau R, et al. Neural processing of spoken words in specific language impairment and dyslexia. Brain 2009;132(Pt 7): 1918–27.

79. Renvall H, Hari R. Auditory cortical responses to speech-like stimuli in dyslexic adults. J Cogn Neurosci 2002;14(5):757–68.

80. Petersen EB, Wöstmann M, Obleser J, et al. Hearing loss impacts neural alpha oscillations under adverse listening conditions. Front Psychol 2015;6. https://doi.org/10.3389/fpsyg.2015.00177.

81. Goswami U. A temporal sampling framework for developmental dyslexia. Trends Cogn Sci 2011; 15(1):3–10.

82. Ahissar M, Lubin Y, Putter-Katz H, et al. Dyslexia and the failure to form a perceptual anchor. Nat Neurosci 2006;9(12):1558–64.

83. Goswami U, Cumming R, Chait M, et al. Perception of filtered speech by children with developmental dyslexia and children with specific language impairments. Front Psychol 2016;7:791.

84. Cumming R, Wilson A, Goswami U. Basic auditory processing and sensitivity to prosodic structure in children with specific language impairments: a new look at a perceptual hypothesis. Front Psychol 2015;6. https://doi.org/10.3389/fpsyg.2015.00972.

85. Lehongre K, Ramus F, Villiermet N, et al. Altered low-γ sampling in auditory cortex accounts for the three main facets of dyslexia. Neuron 2011;72(6):1080–90.

86. Molinaro N, Lizarazu M, Lallier M, et al. Out-of-synchrony speech entrainment in developmental dyslexia. Hum Brain Mapp 2016;37(8):2767–83.

87. Soltész F, Szűcs D, Leong V, et al. Differential entrainment of neuroelectric delta oscillations in developmental dyslexia. PLoS One 2013;8(10): e76608.

88. Leong V, Goswami U. Assessment of rhythmic entrainment at multiple timescales in dyslexia: evidence for disruption to syllable timing. Hearing Res 2014;308:141–61.

89. Chern A, Tillmann B, Vaughan C, et al. New evidence of a rhythmic priming effect that enhances grammaticality judgments in children. J Exp Child Psychol 2018;173:371–9.

90. Bedoin N, Brisseau L, Molinier P, et al. Temporally regular musical primes facilitate subsequent syntax processing in children with specific language impairment. Front Neurosci 2016;10:245.

91. Nozaradan S, Peretz I, Keller PE. Individual differences in rhythmic cortical entrainment correlate with predictive behavior in sensorimotor synchronization. Sci Rep 2016;6(1). https://doi.org/10.1038/srep20612.

92. Cirelli LK, Spinelli C, Nozaradan S, et al. Measuring neural entrainment to beat and meter in infants: effects of music background. Front Neurosci 2016; 10. https://doi.org/10.3389/fnins.2016.00229.

Pediatric Magnetoencephalography in Clinical Practice and Research

Christos Papadelis, PhD[a,b,c],*, Yu-Han Chen, PhD[d]

KEYWORDS

• Source localization • Magnetic source imaging • Epilepsy • Interictal spikes

KEY POINTS

- Magnetoencephalography (MEG) is a noninvasive neuroimaging technique that measures the electromagnetic fields generated by the human brain.
- During an MEG recording, the patient or subject sits comfortably in an armchair that is located inside a magnetically shielded room, which is specially designed to prevent the electromagnetic noise of the environment from overwhelming the weak neural electromagnetic fields.
- The magnetically shielded room is equipped with adjustable lighting and an audiovisual communication system that allows communication with the technical staff seated outside.
- Brain activity is measured by positioning the patient head inside a special helmet that contains magnetic field detection coils, which are inductively coupled to very sensitive magnetic field detection devices, called superconducting quantum interference devices.

INTRODUCTION

Magnetoencephalography (MEG) is a noninvasive neuroimaging technique that measures the electromagnetic fields generated by the human brain. The main sources of these fields are considered to be the postsynaptic currents in the apical dendrites of the cortical pyramidal cells,[1] although action potentials also may be recorded.[2,3] MEG offers an excellent temporal resolution in the range of submilliseconds, that allows even brain activity with high frequencies to be recorded.[4] MEG also offers good spatial resolution via magnetic source imaging (MSI).[5,6] It is most sensitive to the currents that are tangential to the surface of the scalp and blind to magnetic fields produced by radial sources.[7,8]

In clinical practice, MEG is used mostly for the localization of epileptogenic foci in patients with drug-resistant epilepsy undergoing surgery.[9,10] MEG also has become popular for understanding the human brain in both adults and children.[11] During an MEG recording, the patient or subject sits comfortably in an armchair that is located inside a magnetically shielded room, which is specially designed to prevent the electromagnetic noise of the environment from overwhelming the weak neural electromagnetic fields. In several occasions, simultaneous high-density electroencephalogram (EEG) recordings are performed (**Fig. 1**).

[a] Jane and John Justin Neuroscience Center, Cook Children's Health Care System, 1500 Cooper Street, Fort Worth, TX 76104, USA; [b] Department of Pediatrics, TCU and UNTHSC School of Medicine, Fort Worth, TX, USA; [c] Laboratory of Children's Brain Dynamics, Division of Newborn Medicine, Boston Children's Hospital, Harvard Medical School, Boston, MA, USA; [d] Children's Hospital of Philadelphia, CSH115, Department of Radiology, 34th Street and Civic Center Boulevard, Philadelphia, PA 19104, USA
* Corresponding author. Jane and John Justin Neuroscience Center, Cook Children's Health Care System, 1500 Cooper Street, Fort Worth, TX 76104.
E-mail address: christos.papadelis@cookchildrens.org

Neuroimag Clin N Am 30 (2020) 239–248
https://doi.org/10.1016/j.nic.2020.02.002

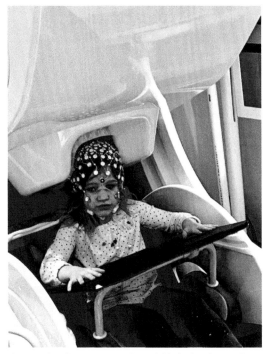

Fig. 1. Simultaneous MEG and high-density EEG recordings from a 4 year-old-girl. Recordings were performed at Cook Children's Health Care System, Fort Worth, Texas.

Recording also can be performed in a supine position when a patient is under sedation or needs to sleep. The magnetically shielded room is equipped with adjustable lighting and an audiovisual communication system that allows communication with the technical staff seated outside. Brain activity is measured by positioning the patient head inside a special helmet that contains magnetic field detection coils, which are inductively coupled to very sensitive magnetic field detection devices, called superconducting quantum interference devices (SQUIDs). In order to operate, SQUID devices must be in an extremely low temperature, close to absolute zero. For this reason, SQUIDs are placed inside a thermo-shielded tank that is filled with liquid helium. Modern MEG systems accommodate a high number of coils up (up to 306).

For decades, MEG was used mostly for measuring the brain activity of adults, and its use in pediatric clinical practice and research was limited. This may be explained by the fact that only adult MEG systems were available in the market. These systems have a fixed-size helmet that is relatively large for pediatric heads, particularly for infants and young children. Yet, several researchers used these systems for pediatric studies (for a review of these studies, see Chen

and colleagues[12]) by placing the children's heads either in the center of an adult MEG helmet or in such a way that the brain area of interest was as close to the sensors as possible. But this placement results in large distances between the active neural generators and the MEG sensors in infants and young children, who have significantly smaller heads compared with the adults. Such a distance leads to less than optimal and sometimes even inadequate signal-to-noise ratio for infant MEG recordings.[13]

This article highlights the benefits that pediatric MEG has to offer to clinical practice and pediatric research, particularly for infants and young children; reviews the existing literature on using adult MEG systems for pediatric use; briefly describes the few pediatric MEG systems currently extant; and draws attention to future directions of research, with focus on the clinical use of MEG for patients with drug-resistant epilepsy.

PEDIATRIC MAGNETOENCEPHALOGRAPHY SYSTEMS

To address the limitations discussed previously, MEG systems specially designed for pediatric use have been developed. These systems are equipped with a helmet having smaller dimensions in order to reduce the distance between the neural generators and MEG sensors. It has been claimed that such a design provides greater sensitivity and spatial resolution compared with adult systems,[14] although these have not yet been quantified. Examples of these systems are (1) the SQUID Array for Reproductive Assessment (SARA) (VSM MedTech, Port Coquitlam, British Columbia, Canada) (Fig. 2A, B)[15] that is being used for fetal and infant MEG recordings; (2) the babySQUID system (Tristan Technologies, San Diego, CA) that has a partial head coverage[10,14] (Fig. 2C); (3) the KIT whole-head system (model PQ1151R) (Yokogawa/KIT, Tokyo, Japan) (Fig. 2D); (4) the Artemis 123 whole-head system (Tristan Technologies, San Diego, CA) (Fig. 2E); and the (5) MagView whole-head system (Tristan Technologies, San Diego, CA)[16] (Fig. 2F). A detailed description of these systems is provided elsewhere.[12]

CLINICAL APPLICATIONS OF PEDIATRIC MAGNETOENCEPHALOGRAPHY

The main clinical application of MEG is in the presurgical evaluation of patients with drug-resistant epilepsy. These patients undergo extensive screening using numerous neuroimaging techniques before their surgery. The goal of this screening is the localization of the epileptogenic

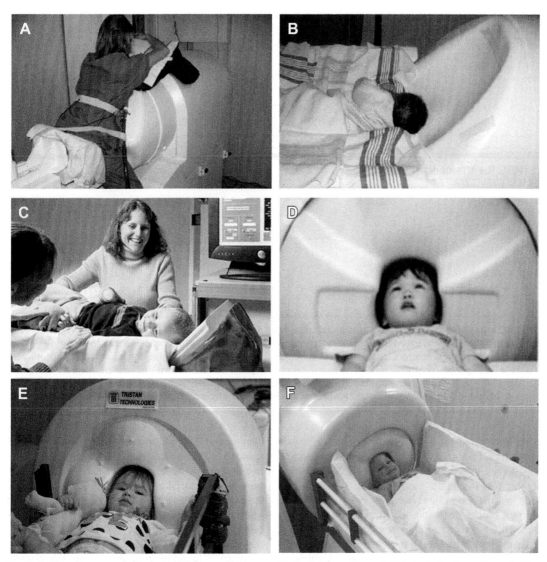

Fig. 2. MEG systems specially designed for pediatric use. (*Adapted from* Chen Y-H, Saby J, Kuschner E, et al. Magnetoencephalography and the infant brain. Neuroimage 2019: 189: 445-458.)

zone, the brain area that is indispensable for the generation of seizures. MEG is used predominantly for the localization of the irritative zone, the brain area that generates interictal epileptiform discharges (IEDs), and for the localization of the eloquent cortex, the cortical areas that are responsible for the different normal functions. It has been shown in 1000 patients with refractory epilepsy that complete resection of the irritative zone localized with MEG is associated with significantly higher chances of achieving seizure freedom in the short term and the long term.[17] These findings show that MEG provides nonredundant information, which significantly contributes to patient selection, focus localization, and ultimately long-term seizure freedom after epilepsy surgery.

The localization of the irritative zone involves the initial identification of the IEDs in the MEG traces, the modeling of the electromagnetic properties of the head and of the sensor array (i.e., the forward model), and finally the estimation of the brain sources, which produced the interictal spikes according to the head model in question (i.e., the inverse problem). MEG source localization also requires coregistration between a patient's anatomy and MEG sensors' locations. MEG spikes are chosen for analysis based on duration (<80 ms), morphology, field map, and lack of associated artifact (Fig. 3). It has been shown that MEG can localize the irritative zone with an accuracy of approximately 15 mm.[18] The forward problem estimates the magnetic field measured outside the

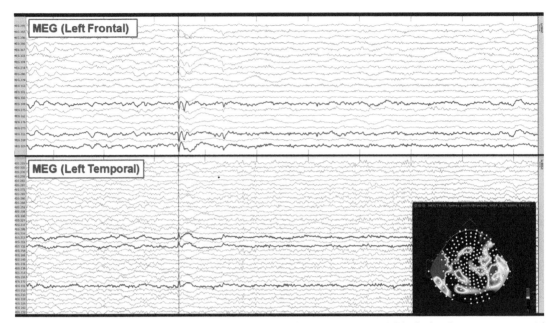

Fig. 3. IEDs in a 4-year-old girl with history of prolonged febrile seizures and febrile focal-onset seizures with gradual impairment of awareness and ultimately motor involvement, including some clonic activity of either side. Display of magnetometers covering the left frontal (*top*) and left temporal (*bottom*) areas. Topography indicates a change of magnetic flux in the left frontotemporal areas. Recordings are performed using the MagView™ system that accommodates 375 magnetometers in a helmet that is specially designed for children up to 4 years old. No sedation was administered during the recording. The recording was performed while the patient was awake.

scalp from a known distribution of neural activity generators using Maxwell's electromagnetic equations. Since the introduction of powerful computers, realistic head models have been used, such as the boundary element model or finite element model, for estimating the forward problem. The inverse problem estimates the most probable neural activity in a child's brain that can explain the MEG signals, which are recorded outside the human's head. The inverse problem does not have a unique solution and requires a priori knowledge about the source generators to constrain the inverse problem solution. Such a constraint assumes that all MEG activity recorded outside the head can be modeled by an infinitesimally small line-current element, the equivalent current dipole (ECD). The ECD is the only validated and approved method for clinical use in the presurgical planning of epilepsy patients.[19–21] It is assumed that each interictal discharge is generated by one ECD. The task is to find the location and direction of this ECD (either at the peak or at the onset of each spike) and overlaid onto the patient's own coregistered brain magnetic resonance image (MRI). This process of modeling the IEDs and overlaying them on patient's MRI often is referred to as magnetic source imaging, MSI. The desirable scenario is a tight cluster of dipoles with similar orientation in a focal brain area ($\geq$20 spikes in a 1-cm area); each of these dipoles represents one interictal discharge (**Fig. 4**). It has been reported that approximately 90% of patients in whom the MEG cluster is completely resected achieve seizure freedom 1 year after resective surgery, whereas only 25% of patients with a partial resection of the MEG cluster attain seizure freedom.[22] In addition, patients are significantly more likely to achieve seizure freedom when the stereotaxic EEG sampling completely covered the MEG clusters. On the other hand, MEG spike sources may have relatively poor correlation with the seizure-onset zone (SOZ), the brain area where seizures are initiated, that is regarded as the best estimator of the epileptogenic zone.[23]

Fig. 5 shows MEG of a pediatric patient with tuberous sclerosis and intractable epilepsy. His MRI showed numerous cortical and subcortical tubers throughout his cerebral hemispheres and numerous subependymal nodules; any of the tubers could have been an epileptic focus. The MEG showed that all his interictal spikes originated from 1 tuber in the right posterolateral temporal lobe. This provided valuable information to the neurosurgeons, guiding them on which tuber to resect, to decrease frequency of seizures.[24]

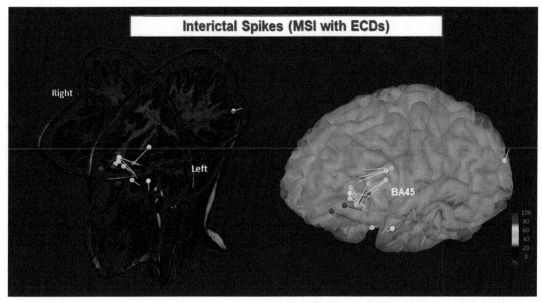

Fig. 4. MSI findings of IEDs identified in Fig. 3. Localization is performed through ECD. Dipoles with goodness-of-fit greater than 60% were considered and displayed. Dipole cluster is localized in the vicinity of Brodmann area 45 (BA45). Right and left indicates left and right hemispheres. Both images depict a 3D representation of the patient's brain (the left is on three slices: axial-coronal-sagittal; the right is on a cortical surface).

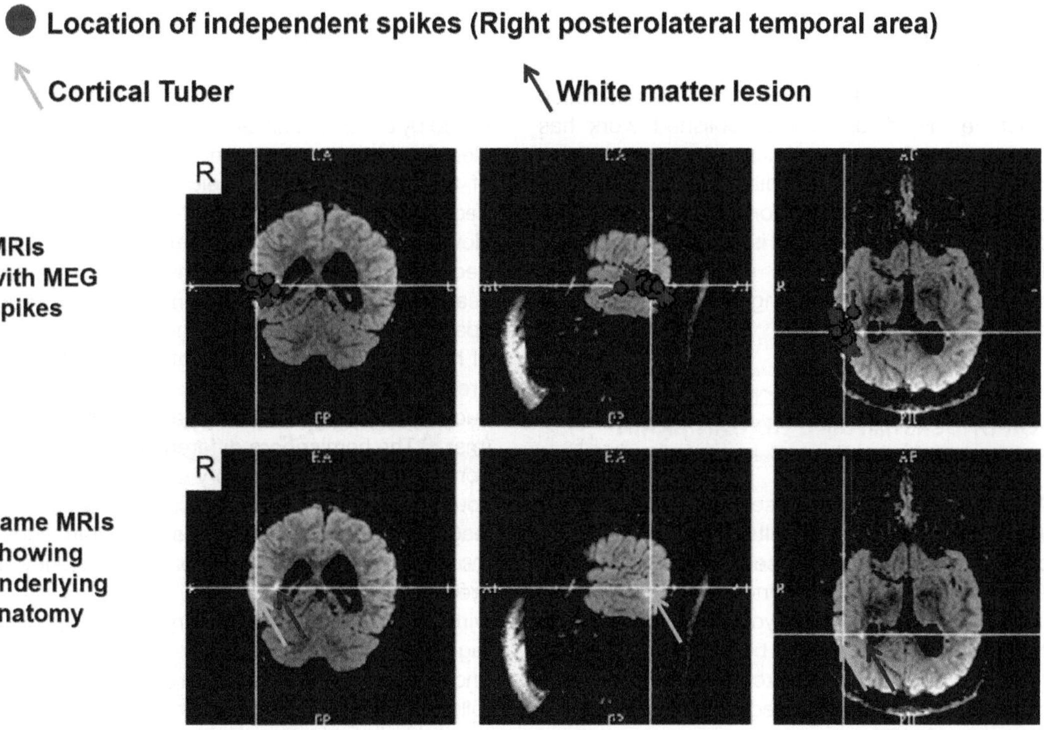

Fig. 5. Pediatric patient with tuberous sclerosis and multiple bilateral cortical and subcortical tubers throughout his cerebrum and with intractable epilepsy. The MEG found 83 interictal spikes over 50 minutes of recording, which all localized to a tuber in the right posterolateral temporal lobe. This aided the neurosurgeons in determining which tuber to resect. (*Courtesy of* Dr R Lee, MD, San Diego, California.)

Several studies have shown that MEG also can be used for the localization of the SOZ, the brain area where the seizures are initiated.[25–27] The SOZ is regarded as a more precise estimator of the epileptogenic zone than the irritative zone. *Ictal* MEG in children demonstrates good concordance with the SOZ, as defined by the current gold standards: intracranial EEG and surgical outcome.[28] Yet, it is challenging to capture a seizure during an MEG scan due to the fact that seizures do not occur all the time and MEG recording time is limited (typically less than an hour) in the clinical setup. Moreover, ictal MEG recordings have low signal-to-noise ratio because ictal activity is obscured from the movement artifact that accompanies the seizure.[29]

Finally, pediatric MEG has been used for the localization of the eloquent cortex in children with refractory epilepsy undergoing surgery. MEG is gaining increasing acceptance for the noninvasive mapping of language[30,31] as well as motor and sensory areas[32–34] compared with other neuroimaging techniques. This mostly is because methods based on electromagnetic measures of brain activity have the advantages of being insensitive to the distortive effects of anatomic lesions on brain microvasculature or metabolism on the developing brain[35] and providing a less intimidating recording environment for younger children.[31] Many of the MEG language studies use similar paradigms, consisting of spoken nouns and a list of target nouns, which must be identified.[36] Little published work has been undertaken on optimizing language protocols specifically for the pediatric population. One of the greatest challenges for MEG with young individuals is to ensure there is minimal movement. To achieve this, scanning procedures need to remain short whilst ensuring adequate signal to noise.

PEDIATRIC MAGNETOENCEPHALOGRAPHY FOR UNDERSTANDING HUMAN BRAIN DEVELOPMENT

Although MEG has been used widely for assessing the brain activity in adults over the past 3 decades, it still is rarely used in developmental research. This has been in part due to the fact that dedicated infant and young children whole-head MEG systems have been developed only recently. In addition to excellent temporal and spatial resolution, discussed previously, the advantages of MEG for measuring neural activity in infants and young children include (1) minimal distortions of volume current caused by incompletely developed fontanels and sutures,[37]

resulting in more accurate source modeling than EEG; (2) head movement compensation methods that correct for use with awake infants during cognitive and sensory tasks; and (3) more accurate source analyses that are possible with age-appropriate MRI templates, mitigating the need for individual MRIs. This section provides an overview of the role of dedicated pediatric MEG systems in developmental cognitive neuroscience research. Given that the critical period of brain development happens early in life, in this section, the review focuses on existing infant MEG studies on basic sensory processes to high-level cognitive processes from birth to 4 years of age. Specifically, studies of the following research fields are discussed: (1) primary auditory processes to simple stimuli; (2) somatosensory processes; (3) visual processes; (4) speech and language processes; and (5) spontaneous resting state brain rhythms.

Auditory Processes in Infants and Young Children

Researchers have utilized MEG to track development of primary sensory auditory responses before and after birth.[15,38–43] Using fetal MEG systems (i.e., SARA), researchers examining auditory evoked responses in fetuses and neonates reported a steady decrease of P2m latency as a function of gestational age. Such studies are unique to MEG, because MEG signals are less distorted by amniotic fluid and layers of skin and muscle. After birth, studies have shown that the latency of the auditory evoked field (AEF) continues to decrease for several years after birth,[44,45] with a slower rate over the first few months of life. Using dedicated whole-head pediatric MEG systems, researchers were able to examine activity in source space and separately examine the development of hemispheric lateralization of AEF. In older children, studies have shown earlier right than left auditory response latency at 50 milliseconds (ms).[46] The hemisphere differences in the maturation of left and right auditory cortex in infants and young children still remain unclear. Edgar and colleagues[44] showed that across children ages 6 months to 59 months, auditory P2m latency decreases at a rate of approximately 0.6 ms/mo, with right hemisphere auditory encoding advantages observed only under more demanding encoding conditions. Longitudinal studies following children from infancy through toddlerhood to school age are needed to better understand the hemisphere maturation rate of infant and young child AEF and how it is associated with later left hemisphere lateralization for word processing that emerges during reading acquisition.[44] Looking to the future, multimodal imaging studies in pediatric populations will provide direct examination of associations between brain neural function and brain structure to better understand the mechanisms that support maturation of different brain regions and the development of language. As a first step, however, given the limitation and lower success rate of obtaining structural or functional MRI in pediatric populations, MEG is the most optimal neuroimaging modality to measure whole-brain neural networks associated with basic and high-level cognitive processes in children.

Somatosensory Processes in Infants and Young Children

Research examining primary/secondary somatosensory cortical activity in children typically employ painless pneumatic tactile stimuli.[33,34] Somatosensory evoked fields (SEFs) in newborns traditionally were measured in response to tactile stimulation applied to the fingertip of sleeping infants positioned against one side of a conventional adult-sized MEG helmet.[47-51] Infant SEFs were observed as one broad and slower deflection approximately 60 ms poststimulus, localized in the contralateral primary somatosensory cortex (SI). In adult literature, SEFs were characterized as two deflections from SI. The morphology differences of SEFs between infants and adults might be due to possible GABAergic inhibitory processes, which are not yet maturing in infants.[52] Regarding clinical application of infant SEFs, several studies have suggested that SEFs localized in secondary somatosensory cortex (SII), peaking at approximately 200 ms poststimulus, may be a prognostic brain marker for predicting outcome in preterm infants[53,54] or infants born with prenatal drug exposure.[55] Other studies have focused on developmental changes of sensorimotor brain rhythms, such as mu-rhythm peak frequency,[52,53] as well as functional connectivity measures of sensorimotor neural network.

Visual Processes in Infants and Young Children

Few studies have used MEG to study primary visual evoked fields (VEFs) or evoked responses or brain responses to social or face stimuli in young children. Using a train of light flashes, studies have shown decreased VEFs to successive light flashes as a sign of habituation of visual responses in fetuses and newborns.[43,56] Although neuroimaging studies examining visual processes or socio-cognitive processes using visual stimuli (e.g., face) have been done in preschool-aged or school-aged children,[57,58] MEG studies examining how infants process social visual stimuli have not yet been conducted.

Speech and Language Processes in Infants

Most of the MEG studies examining how language is processed during the first year of life have focused on localizing language-related brain regions beyond primary auditory cortex.[59-63] Compared with other neuroimaging techniques, MEG is unique in that it can be used to study higher-level cognitive processes (e.g., language processes) throughout the whole brain in awake infants and young children. Using distributed source modeling (for example, minimum norm estimation[8]), Broca area and cerebellum have been found to be involved in passive encoding speech sounds as well as speech production in addition to auditory cortex.[60,61] A growing literature of bilingual processes in infants also showed that prefrontal and orbitofrontal areas are involved during passive listening of speech sounds in bilingual but not monolingual infants, suggesting that dual language exposure during infancy may be related to the development of executive function skills later in life.[64-66]

Resting-State Brain Rhythms in Infants and Young Children

Characterizing spontaneous brain rhythms in awake infants and young children is challenging. Characteristics of low-frequency brain rhythms also have been studied as potential indicators of brain pathology in adult literature. As such, studies characterizing slow rhythms early in life can be used as a potential brain marker for infants at risk for developmental disorder. For example, Sanjuan and colleagues[67] showed associations between theta power and maternal stress in infants, suggesting a delay in cortical maturation in infants born to mothers with posttraumatic stress disorder.

FUTURE DIRECTIONS

Efficacy and safety of pediatric epilepsy surgery have been significantly improved over the past decades.[68] Only a third of pediatric surgical candidates, however, proceed to surgery within 2 years of onset, despite this onset having occurred at less than 2 years of age in 60% of the children.[69,70] Recent progress in pediatric MEG has provided a comprehensive surgical management for these patients,[10,71] although its use is limited. Application of MEG in young children with epilepsy will accelerate during the coming years, as different types of pediatric whole-head MEG systems and more advanced data analysis methods become available to researchers and clinicians. These advances will lead to greater use of MEG as a complement to clinical EEG, with improved noninvasive delineation of the epileptogenic zone. Research examining brain neural activity in pediatric populations using EEG is sizable, and studies examining patterns of brain blood flow in infants using functional MRI are increasingly prominent. As this review indicates, MEG is a promising noninvasive technology for studying infant and young children's brains, offering complementary information for understanding the development of brain function beyond brain structure in pediatric populations, especially in infants and young children. Recent advances in MEG analyses, particularly in the use of age-matched MRI templates instead of individual MRIs, will facilitate analyses of brain function in source space, thereby providing greater potential to study brain networks and functional connectivity in pediatric MEG research. With emerging hardware as well as analysis pipelines dedicated specifically to pediatric populations that provides necessary sensitivity, future pediatric MEG research and clinical studies likely will apply distributed source localization to examine activity throughout the brain, and thus facilitate studies of local and long-range functional connectivity. Longitudinal as well as cross-sectional studies are needed to evaluate the developmental trajectory (maturation) of neural activity in the first few years of life. It is expected that departures from neurotypical trajectories will offer early detection and prognosis insights in infants and toddlers at risk for neurodevelopmental disorders, thus paving the way for early targeted interventions.

SUMMARY

During the past 10 years, MEG has become increasingly useful for the presurgical delineation of epileptogenic zones and eloquent cortex in both lesional and nonlesional pediatric cases. Several studies also have used pediatric MEG to study brain development, particularly at early years of life during critical periods. Application of MEG in pediatric epilepsy and research of human development will accelerate during the coming years as different types of pediatric whole-head MEG systems and more advanced data analysis methods become available to researchers and clinicians.

DISCLOSURES

This study was supported by the National Institute of Neurological Disorders & Stroke (RO1NS104116-01A1, PI: C. Papadelis; and R21NS101373-01A1, PIs: C. Papadelis and S. Stufflebeam).

REFERENCES

1. Murakami S, Okada Y. Contributions of principal neocortical neurons to magnetoencephalography and electroencephalography signals. J Physiol 2006;575(Pt 3):925–36.
2. Kimura T, Ozaki I, Hashimoto I. Impulse propagation along thalamocortical fibers can be detected magnetically outside the human brain. J Neurosci 2008;28(47):12535–8.
3. Papadelis C, Leonardelli E, Staudt M, et al. Can magnetoencephalography track the afferent information flow along white matter thalamo-cortical fibers? Neuroimage 2012;60(2):1092–105.
4. Papadelis C, Tamilia E, Stufflebeam S, et al. Interictal high frequency oscillations detected with simultaneous magnetoencephalography and electroencephalography as biomarker of pediatric epilepsy. J Vis Exp 2016;(118):e54883.
5. Miller GA, Elbert T, Sutton BP, et al. Innovative clinical assessment technologies: challenges and opportunities in neuroimaging. Psychol Assess 2007; 19:58–73.
6. Papadelis C, Poghosyan V, Fenwick PB, et al. MEG's ability to localise accurately weak transient neural sources. Clin Neurophysiol 2009;120:1958–70.
7. Cohen D, Hosaka H. Part II: magnetic field produced by a current dipole. J Electrocardiol 1976; 9(4):409–17.
8. Hämäläinen MS, Hari R, Ilmoniemi RJ, et al. Magnetoencephalography—theory, instrumentation, and applications to noninvasive studies of the working human brain. Rev Mod Phys 1993;65:413–97.
9. Englot DJ, Ouyang D, Garcia PA, et al. Epilepsy surgery trends in the United States, 1990–2008. Neurology 2012;78:1200–6.
10. Papadelis C, Harini C, Ahtam B, et al. Current and emerging potential for magnetoencephalography in pediatric epilepsy. J Pediatr Epilepsy 2013;2:73–85.
11. Baillet S. Magnetoencephalography for brain electrophysiology and imaging. Nat Neurosci 2017;20: 327–39.
12. Chen Y-H, Saby J, Kuschner E, et al. Magnetoencephalography and the infant brain. Neuroimage 2019;189:445–58.
13. Gaetz W, Otsubo H, Pang EW. Magnetoencephalography for clinical pediatrics: the effect of head positioning on measurement of somatosensory-evoked fields. Clin Neurophysiol 2008;119:1923–33.

14. Okada Y, Pratt K, Atwood C, et al. BabySQUID: a mobile, high-resolution multichannel magnetoencephalography system for neonatal brain assessment. Rev Sci Instrum 2006;77:024301.

15. Holst M, Eswaran H, Lowery C, et al. Development of auditory evoked fields in human fetuses and newborns: a longitudinal MEG study. Clin Neurophysiol 2005;116:1949–55.

16. Okada Y, Hamalainen M, Pratt K, et al. BabyMEG: a whole-head pediatric magnetoencephalography system for human brain development research. Rev Sci Instrum 2016;87:094301.

17. Rampp S, Stefan H, Wu X, et al. Magnetoencephalography for epileptic focus localization in a series of 1000 cases. Brain 2019;142(10):3059–71.

18. Tamilia E, AlHilani M, Tanaka N, et al. Assessing the localization accuracy and clinical utility of electric and magnetic source imaging in children with epilepsy. Clin Neurophysiol 2019;130(4):491–504.

19. Barth DS, Sutherling W, Engel J, et al. Neuromagnetic localization of epileptiform spike activity in the human brain. Science 1982;218(4575):891–4.

20. Knowlton RC, Laxer KD, Aminoff MJ, et al. Magnetoencephalography in partial epilepsy: clinical yield and localization accuracy. Ann Neurol 1997;42(4):622–31.

21. Stefan H, Hummel C, Scheler G, et al. Magnetic brain source imaging of focal epileptic activity: a synopsis of 455 cases. Brain 2003;126(11):2396–405.

22. Murakami H, Wang ZI, Marashly A, et al. Correlating magnetoencephalography to stereoelectroencephalography in patients undergoing epilepsy surgery. Brain 2016;139(11):2935–47.

23. Kim D, Joo EY, Seo DW, et al. Accuracy of MEG in localizing irritative zone and seizure onset zone: quantitative comparison between MEG and intracranial EEG. Epilepsy Res 2016;127:291–301.

24. Hunold A, Haueisen J, Ahtam B, et al. Localization of the epileptogenic foci in tuberous sclerosis complex: a pediatric case report. Front Hum Neurosci 2014;8:175.

25. Assaf BA, Karkar KM, Laxer KD, et al. Ictal magnetoencephalography in temporal and extratemporal lobe epilepsy. Epilepsia 2003;44(10):1320–7.

26. Eliashiv DS, Elsas SM, Squires K, et al. Ictal magnetic source imaging as a localizing tool in partial epilepsy. Neurology 2002;59(10):1600–10.

27. Shiraishi H, Watanabe Y, Watanabe M, et al. Interictal and ictal magnetoencephalographic study in patients with medial frontal lobe epilepsy. Epilepsia 2001;42(7):875–82.

28. Fujiwara H, Greiner HM, Hemasilpin N, et al. Ictal MEG onset source localization compared to intracranial EEG and outcome: improved epilepsy presurgical evaluation in pediatrics. Epilepsy Res 2012;99(3):214–24.

29. Medvedovsky M, Taulu S, Gaily E, et al. Sensitivity and specificity of seizure-onset zone estimation by ictal magnetoencephalography. Epilepsia 2012;53(9):1649–57.

30. Foley E, Cross JH, Thai NJ, et al. MEG assessment of expressive language in children evaluated for epilepsy surgery. Brain Topogr 2019;32(3):492–503.

31. Pang EW, Wang F, Malone M, et al. Localization of Brocàs area using verb generation tasks in the MEG: Validation against fMRI. Neurosci Lett 2011;490:215–9.

32. Castillo EM, Simos PG, Wheless JW, et al. Integrating sensory and motor mapping in a comprehensive MEG protocol: clinical validity and replicability. Neuroimage 2004;21(3):973–83.

33. Papadelis C, Ahtam B, Nazarova M, et al. Cortical somatosensory reorganization in children with spastic cerebral palsy: a multimodal neuroimaging study. Front Hum Neurosci 2014;8:725.

34. Papadelis C, Butler EE, Rubenstein M, et al. Reorganization of the somatosensory cortex in hemiplegic cerebral palsy associated with impaired sensory tracts. Neuroimage Clin 2017;17:198–212.

35. Demonet JF, Thierry G, Cardebat D. Renewal of the neurophysiology of language: Functional neuroimaging. Physiol Rev 2005;85:49–95.

36. Tsigka S, Papadelis C, Braun C, et al. Distinguishable neural correlates of verbs and nouns: a MEG study on homonyms. Neuropsychologia 2014;54:87–97.

37. Lew S, Sliva DD, Choe MS, et al. Effects of sutures and fontanels on MEG and EEG source analysis in a realistic infant head model. Neuroimage 2013;76:282–93.

38. Draganova R, Eswaran H, Murphy P, et al. Serial magnetoencephalographic study of fetal and newborn auditory discriminative evoked responses. Early Hum Dev 2007;83:199–207.

39. Draganova R, Eswaran H, Murphy P, et al. Sound frequency change detection in fetuses and newborns, a magnetoencephalographic study. Neuroimage 2005;28:354–61.

40. Govindan RB, Wilson JD, Preissl H, et al. An objective assessment of fetal and neonatal auditory evoked responses. Neuroimage 2008;43:521–7.

41. Hartkopf J, Schleger F, Weiss M, et al. Neuromagnetic signatures of syllable processing in fetuses and infants provide no evidence for habituation. Early Hum Dev 2016;100:61–6.

42. Lengle JM, Chen M, Wakai RT. Improved neuromagnetic detection of fetal and neonatal auditory evoked responses. Clin Neurophysiol 2001;112:785–92.

43. Sheridan CJ, Preissl H, Siegel ER, et al. Neonatal and fetal response decrement of evoked responses: a MEG study. Clin Neurophysiol 2008;119:796–804.

44. Edgar JC, Murray R, Kuschner ES, et al. The maturation of auditory responses in infants and young children: a cross-sectional study from 6 to 59 months. Front Neuroanat 2015;9:131.

45. Stephen JM, Hill DE, Peters A, et al. Development of auditory evoked responses in normally developing preschool children and children with autism spectrum disorder. Dev Neurosci 2017;39:430–41.

46. Gomes H, Dunn M, RitterW, et al. Spatiotemporal maturation of the central and lateral N1 components to tones. Brain Res Dev Brain Res 2001;129(2): 147–55.

47. Lauronen L, Nevalainen P, Wikstrom H, et al. Immaturity of somatosensory cortical processing in human newborns. Neuroimage 2006;33:195–203.

48. Nevalainen P, Lauronen L, Sambeth A, et al. Somatosensory evoked magnetic fields from the primary and secondary somatosensory cortices in healthy newborns. Neuroimage 2008;40:738–45.

49. Nevalainen P, Pihko E, Metsaranta M, et al. Evoked magnetic fields from primary and secondary somatosensory cortices: a reliable tool for assessment of cortical processing in the neonatal period. Clin Neurophysiol 2012;123:2377–83.

50. Pihko E, Lauronen L. Somatosensory processing in healthy newborns. Exp Neurol 2004;190(Suppl 1): S2–7.

51. Pihko E, Nevalainen P, Stephen J, et al. Maturation of somatosensory cortical processing from birth to adulthood revealed by magnetoencephalography. Clin Neurophysiol 2009;120:1552–61.

52. Nevalainen P, Lauronen L, Pihko E. Development of human somatosensory cortical functions - what have we learned from magnetoencephalography: a review. Front Hum Neurosci 2014;8:158.

53. Nevalainen P, Rahkonen P, Pihko E, et al. Evaluation of somatosensory cortical processing in extremely preterm infants at term with MEG and EEG. Clin Neurophysiol 2015;126:275–83.

54. Rahkonen P, Nevalainen P, Lauronen L, et al. Cortical somatosensory processing measured by magnetoencephalography predicts neurodevelopment in extremely low-gestational-age infants. Pediatr Res 2013;73:763–71.

55. Kivisto K, Nevalainen P, Lauronen L, et al. Somatosensory and auditory processing in opioid-exposed newborns with neonatal abstinence syndrome: a magnetoencephalographic approach. J Matern Fetal Neonatal Med 2015;28:2015–9.

56. Matuz T, Govindan RB, Preissl H, et al. Habituation of visual evoked responses in neonates and fetuses: a MEG study. Dev Cogn Neurosci 2012;2:303–16.

57. He W, Brock J, Johnson BW. Face-sensitive brain responses measured from a four-year-old child with a custom-sized child MEG system. J Neurosci Methods 2014;222:213–7.

58. Taylor MJ, Donner EJ, Pang EW. fMRI and MEG in the study of typical and atypical cognitive development. Neurophysiol Clin 2012;42:19–25.

59. Ferjan Ramirez N, Ramirez RR, Clarke M, et al. Speech discrimination in 11-month-old bilingual and monolingual infants: a magnetoencephalography study. Dev Sci 2017;20. https://doi.org/10.1111/desc.12427.

60. Imada T, Zhang Y, Cheour M, et al. Infant speech perception activates Broca's area: a developmental magnetoencephalography study. Neuroreport 2006;17:957–62.

61. Kuhl PK, Ramirez RR, Bosseler A, et al. Infants' brain responses to speech suggest analysis by synthesis. Proc Natl Acad Sci U S A 2014;111: 11238–45.

62. Travis KE, Leonard MK, Brown TT, et al. Spatiotemporal neural dynamics of word understanding in 12- to 18-month-old-infants. Cereb Cortex 2011;21: 1832–9.

63. Zhao TC, Kuhl PK. Musical intervention enhances infants' neural processing of temporal structure in music and speech. Proc Natl Acad Sci U S A 2016;113: 5212–7.

64. Estes KG, Hay JF. Flexibility in bilingual infants' word learning. Child Dev 2015;86:1371–85.

65. Kovacs AM, Mehler J. Cognitive gains in 7-month-old bilingual infants. Proc Natl Acad Sci U S A 2009;106:6556–60.

66. Kovacs AM, Mehler J. Flexible learning of multiple speech structures in bilingual infants. Science 2009;325:611–2.

67. Sanjuan PM, Poremba C, Flynn LR, et al. Association between theta power in 6-month old infants at rest and maternal PTSD severity: a pilot study. Neurosci Lett 2016;630:120–6.

68. Langfitt JT, Holloway RG, McDermott MP, et al. Health care costs decline after successful epilepsy surgery. Neurology 2007;68(16):1290–8.

69. Harvey AS, Cross JH, Shinnar S, et al. Defining the spectrum of international practice in pediatric epilepsy surgery patients. Epilepsia 2008;49(1): 146–55.

70. Ryvlin P, Cross JH, Rheims S. Epilepsy surgery in children and adults. Lancet Neurol 2014;13(11): 1114–26.

71. Guan J, Karsy M, Ducis K, et al. Surgical strategies for pediatric epilepsy. Transl Pediatr 2016;5(2): 55–66.

Merging Magnetoencephalography into Epilepsy Presurgical Work-up Under the Framework of Multimodal Integration

Joon Yul Choi, PhD, Zhong Irene Wang, PhD*

KEYWORDS

- MEG • Multimodal • Epilepsy • Presurgical evaluation • ICEEG • SEEG

KEY POINTS

- Success of epilepsy surgery is highly dependent on a solid presurgical hypothesis after careful analyses of preoperative noninvasive tests, for which multimodal image integration is important.
- Assessing concordance between MEG and other tests can provide essential information for planning of intracranial EEG implantation, particularly stereo-EEG.
- Multimodal integration of MEG also benefits interpretation of intracranial EEG data, planning of final resection, and addressing surgical failures.

INTRODUCTION

Approximately 30% of epilepsy patients are drug-refractory and suffer from incapacitating seizures with worsened quality of life. For patients with drug-refractory focal epilepsy, surgery is currently their best hope for seizure control.[1] Beyond reduction of seizures, simulation models suggest that epilepsy surgery increases life expectancy by a mean of 5 years and quality-adjusted life expectancy by 7.5 years.[2] Patients with difficult-to-localize epilepsy generally need to undergo substantial presurgical noninvasive testing, which may include history, seizure semiology, 3-T MR imaging (MRI), scalp video-electroencephalogram (EEG), PET, ictal single-photon emission computed tomography (SPECT), magnetoencephalography (MEG), functional MRI, neuropsychological testing, and WADA test (also known as the intracarotid sodium amobarbital

procedure). Intracranial EEG (ICEEG) is frequently required for further localization of the seizure onset zone when noninvasive tests could not lead to a conclusive surgical strategy.[3] The success of ICEEG and subsequent surgery is highly dependent on a solid presurgical hypothesis that is generated after careful analyses of the noninvasive tests, and integrating localization information from various preoperative modalities is essential for this process.

Multimodal image integration, also known as coregistration or fusion, refers to the procedure that puts together imaging data from multiple sources into the same space (the patient's individual space) by a computerized registration process. The inputs to multimodal image integration typically include test data such as MRI, PET and SPECT, exported as DICOM files or volume files; localization results from EEG and/or MEG are stored in more variable formats depending on the

Epilepsy Center, Neurological Institute, Cleveland Clinic, Desk S51, 9500 Euclid Avenue, Cleveland, OH 44195, USA
* Corresponding author.
E-mail address: wangi2@ccf.org

Neuroimag Clin N Am 30 (2020) 249–259
https://doi.org/10.1016/j.nic.2020.01.005

source localization software, and using these results as inputs to multimodal integration is more challenging. Although results from each test can be reviewed separately within each vendor platform, and an experienced epileptologist/surgeon/neuroradiologist can mentally fuse the localization results together, the multimodal image integration process offers a more straightforward and convenient solution. This is especially helpful when there is marked difference of head position in between tests and when anatomic landmarks are difficult to find because of different imaging planes. This article first introduces the methodology of multimodal image integration for epilepsy presurgical evaluation, with the focus on integration of MEG. Next we summarize the multifaceted aspects where this integration process benefits planning of ICEEG and resective surgery. Special emphasis is given to implications for stereo-EEG (SEEG), where imaging guidance from multimodal integration is crucial.

METHODOLOGY OVERVIEW

Although the exact platform used depends on local expertise, multimodal image integration is typically built as a step-by-step process by which each new modality is coregistered with the base anatomic image (typically a three-dimensional [3D] T1-weighted MR image), and display settings are adjusted for image overlay. The final multimodal image is visualized with two-dimensional (2D) view or 3D volume rendering; brain surface is displayed with volumes or clusters representing different modalities. The multimodal platform preferably allows for interaction from the users, including alteration of transparency, rotation of the image/volume in any plane, and changing the contrast and brightness of the images for best visualization.

Preimplantation Image Integration

Fig. 1 illustrates an example of multiple integrated modalities for a patient undergoing presurgical noninvasive evaluation at the Cleveland Clinic Epilepsy Center. The workflow was based on Food and Drug Administration–approved software platform Curry 7 (Compumedics Neuroscan, Hamburg, Germany). Overall, the data structure was organized as databases, with each modality stored as one data folder/file within the database. When each modality was imported for the first time, an initialization process was needed to set the parameters, followed by image coregistration. The 3D T1-weighted Magnetization Prepared Rapid Acquisition with Gradient Echo (MPRAGE) volumetric was used as the base image volume. Other sequences of different MRI contrasts,

such as FLAIR, T2-weighted images, were coregistered to the T1-weighted base image by automated full-volume registration (maximization of mutual information). Similarly, the attenuation-corrected fluorodeoxyglucose (FDG)-PET images were coregistered with the T1-weighted base image, displayed with transparency settings optimized for viewing of PET fused with MRI. SPECT interictal image was subtracted from the ictal image and analyzed following methodology of SISCOM.[4] This analysis yielded the subtracted z score image volume with the MRI volume to which it was coregistered. We coregistered this MRI volume to the T1-weighted base image and use the same transformation matrix for the subtracted z score image. Spontaneous MEG data were recorded from a 306-channel whole-head MEG system (Elekta, Helsinki, Finland) and source localization analysis for MEG was performed by the vendor NeuroMag software using single equivalent current dipole model.[5] The final result was represented by one or several clusters of dipoles superimposed on the patient's MRI. We exported the location of the MEG dipoles by printing them as high-intensity points on the MRI. The MRI after the printing process were then coregistered to the T1-weighted base image. The high-intensity points representing the dipole locations were then segmented and their 3D coordinates were saved as a list of "localize points," and visualized in conjunction with all the other data. To visualize vasculature, computed tomography (CT) angiography and magnetic resonance angiography images were registered to the T1-weighted base image; image contrast was adjusted so that when overlaid, major vessels were visible. The outputs of functional MRI scan were statistical maps superimposed on MPRAGE images, which were imported and coregistered to the T1-weighted base volume. Fig. 1 illustrates T1-weighted MRI, FDG-PET, SPECT SISCOM, MEG, axial FLAIR, and axial T2-weighted TSE images from the same patient; after the coregistration was completed, the green cursor was synchronized on all the modalities and can be placed anywhere to examine any region of interest. For example, when examining the tight MEG cluster in the left centroparietal region (cursor location in Fig. 1), concordance with SISCOM hyperperfusion was seen, suggesting that this region could be a legitimate target for further exploration (because of its involvement on MEG and SPECT).

A detailed cortical surface rendering was generated by Freesurfer (Martinos Center for Biomedical Imaging, http://www.nmr.mgh.harvard.edu/) and then imported to Curry. The pial surface files

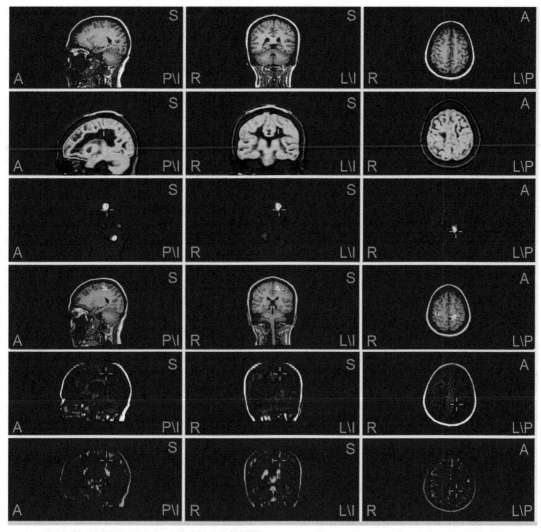

Fig. 1. Illustration of multimodality image integration from a patient undergoing noninvasive presurgical evaluation. Rows from top to bottom: 3D T1-weighted MRI, fluorodeoxyglucose-PET, SPECT SISCOM (z score = 2), MEG (dipole locations), 2D axial FLAIR and 2D axial T2-weighted TSE images. *Green cursor* is centered on the tight MEG cluster in the left centroparietal region and the corresponding location is shown on all the other modalities by green cursors. A, anterior; I, inferior; L, left; P, posterior; R, right; S, superior.

generated by Freesurfer were first transformed to Curry surface format, and then spatially coregistered with the T1-weighted base image. Once this coregistration is complete, each point on the cortical surface was linked to the coronal, axial, and sagittal views of the T1-weighted image and all other images coregistered to it, allowing for visualization of the cortical surface with all the other noninvasive data (example in **Fig. 8**A). A Talairach grid was defined based on anterior commissure, posterior commissure, and midsagittal points identified on the T1-weighted base image; then the boundary box of the brain was delineated on the sagittal view (anterior, posterior, superior, and inferior boundaries) and axial view

(lateral boundaries). When defined, the Talairach grid is shown on 2D and 3D views (**Fig. 2**).

Stereo-EEG Trajectory Planning

After all the images were fused and Talairach coordinates defined, trajectories of SEEG are planned based on any chosen modality of particular relevance to the case. An entry point and a target point were defined for each electrode, and the trajectories were created as a straight line connecting these two points. The Talairach grid was used as a reference to facilitate the definition of the entry and target points. **Fig. 3** illustrates four different cases in which trajectories were planned to target

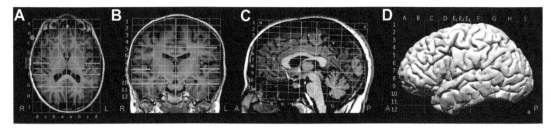

Fig. 2. Illustration of Talairach grid defined based on anterior commissure (AC), posterior commissure (PC), and midsagittal (MS) points identified on the 3D T1-weighted base image. (*A–C*) 2D overlay of the Talairach grid on coronal, axial, and sagittal MRI. (*D*) 3D overlay of the Talairach grid on cortical surface. *Green lines* indicate electrode trajectories. A, anterior; L, left; P, posterior; R, right.

a tight MEG cluster (see **Fig. 3**A), SPECT hyperperfusion regions for assessment of seizure onset/propagation (see **Fig. 3**B), and PET hypometabolism extent (see **Fig. 3**C). To ensure the safety of implantation, CT angiography and magnetic resonance angiography images are used to fine-tune the planned trajectories to avoid collision of the electrode paths with major vessels, particularly at the entry points (see **Fig. 3**D). All planned trajectories can then be exported on top of the T1-weighted MRI DICOM images, and incorporated into the neuronavigation systems (eg, ROSA [Medtech, Montpellier, France] and Brainlab [Brainlab, Feldkirchen, Germany]) for implanting the electrodes in the operating room.

Postimplantation Reconstruction and Resection Planning

The CT images taken immediately after the ICEEG implantation were used to indicate the location of the electrodes that were actually implanted. After fusing with the T1-weighted base image, all electrode contacts were segmented from the CT and stored as a list of localize points with coordinates for the electrode contacts, as shown in **Fig. 4**. Because the preimplantation noninvasive modalities, such as MRI, PET, SISCOM, and MEG, were all registered to the same space of the T1-weighted base image, and the postimplantation CT image was also coregistered to the same space, direct comparison between the SEEG data and the noninvasive evaluation data was possible. **Fig. 5** illustrates a case where the SEEG contacts involved at ictal onset "triangulated" the MEG cluster, showing excellent sublobar concordance. Such direct comparison can often shed light on the interpretation of SEEG data.

Because of MRI safety precautions for patients with implanted intracranial electrodes, postimplantation MRI is often not performed. The electrode location reconstruction is typically based on preimplantation MRI and postimplantation CT.

It is therefore important to consider brain "sagging" in the case of open-dura surgery (eg, subdural grid implantation), that is, the surface of the brain has moved inward, as compared with the preoperative intact brain. As measured by a prior study using 3D electrode models created with post-grid CT and MRI combined with intraoperative navigational measures of electrode positions, statistically significant shift can occur in 50% of patients, with overall magnitude differences in electrode positions averaging about 7 mm.[6] Therefore, when high precision is required, transformation to "morph" the depressed brain back to its preoperative state is necessary. This issue, however, has lesser effect on clinical practice nowadays because of an increasing number/percentage of SEEG implantation, for which the dura is not open and brain sagging is rarely seen.

Planning of the resection on the multimodal integration platform is also possible after considering noninvasive and invasive data. As shown in **Fig. 6**, the proposed resection area is interactively drawn on the 3D T1-weighted base MRI (on 2D coronal, axial, and sagittal views), and can also be segmented as voxel mesh shown in 3D view together with the cortical surface. As a last step, the proposed resection area could be exported as a high-intensity area printed on MRI DICOMs and imported to the neuronavigation system to guide resection. At the end of the operation, the extent of the proposed resection could be confirmed with an intraoperative MRI coregistered to the preoperative T1-weighted MRI with the proposed resection overlaid.

CLINICAL VALUE

The essence for multimodal presurgical evaluation is to generate, inform, dispute, or add to the electroclinical hypothesis. Putting together the noninvasive data in the same space assists the assessment of whether there is adequate overlap between the cortical regions indicated by the

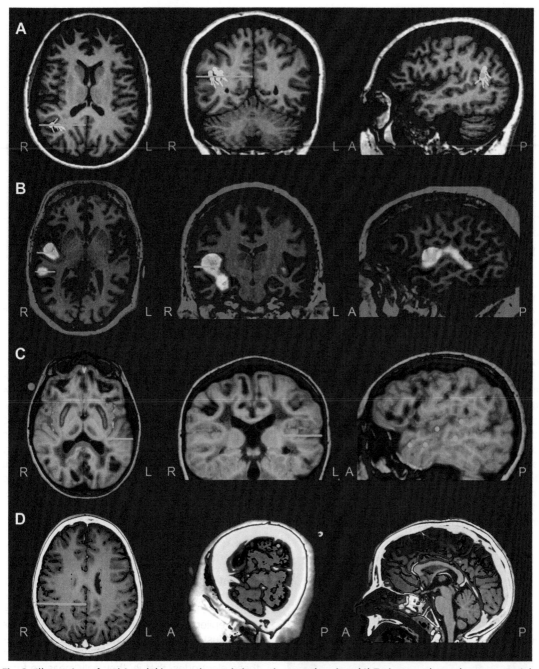

Fig. 3. Illustration of multimodal integration assisting trajectory planning. (*A*) Trajectory planned to target a tight MEG cluster. (*B*) Trajectories planned to target interconnected SPECT hyperperfusion regions. (*C*) Trajectories planned to target PET hypometabolism extent. (*D*) CT angiography images used to fine-tune the planned trajectories to avoid major vessels, particularly at the entry point (*left*, axial view of CT angiography thresholded and overlaid on MRI; *middle*, sagittal view of the overlay showing entry point of the trajectory; *right*, sagittal view of the overlay showing target point of the trajectory). A, anterior; L, left; P, posterior; R, right.

noninvasive test battery, or if any network hypothesis can be generated to explain the data at hand. This is especially pertinent with SEEG implantation for deep focus, or cases where the epileptogenic zone had no clear borders. The use of multimodal image integration has shown demonstrated value for the presurgical evaluation of epilepsy patients. Nowell and colleagues[7] reported substantial changes in ICEEG after presenting multimodality image integration data. The study compared the

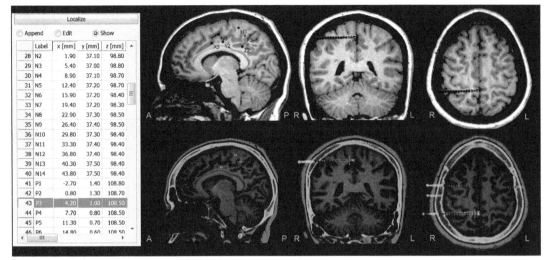

Fig. 4. Post-SEEG-implantation CT images coregistered with the T1-weighted base image, with all the electrode contacts segmented from the CT (center of highest intensity) and stored as a list of localize points with coordinates for the electrode contacts. *Blue spheres* indicate extracted electrode contacts. *Red contact* indicates the current electrode contact (highlighted from the list of localize points), the location of which is synchronized on the MRI and CT. A, anterior; L, left; P, posterior; R, right.

decisions made by the multidisciplinary team on the strategy and the actual trajectory planning of ICEEG before and after multimodal image integration data was shown. In the 44 patients studied, disclosure of the multimodality image integration data led to a change in surgical strategy in about one-third, including addition and subtraction of electrodes, addition of grids, and going directly to resection. Although MEG was not performed in every case, the authors reported two instances (2/15) where surgical strategies were altered by integrating MEG results. In terms of detailed

surgical/trajectory planning, 35 (81%) of 43 showed a change after disclosure of 3D multimodal image integration data. Most of these changes occurred in patients with SEEG and not for subdural grid implantation in terms of grid sizing and positioning. Our experience echoes this study, in that SEEG benefits most sustainably from multimodal image integration, because it heavily depends on imaging guidance. Next we discuss the most pertinent scenarios in terms of the value of integrating MEG.

Importance of Prospective Sampling of Magnetoencephalography-Indicated Regions

Accurate integration of MEG results into surgical planning is most relevant when single or multiple tight MEG clusters are present, indicating potential active epileptogenic sources. Precise targeting of these clusters with intracranial electrodes is paramount because of the "tunnel vision" nature of these electrodes, that is, they only measure focal excitation of neuron within a certain distance. Kakisaka and colleagues[8] reported a strong quadratic fall-off relationship between the amplitude of spikes seen on SEEG and distance between SEEG spikes and MEG spikes (R^2 >0.9); with a distance between SEEG and MEG cluster being 10 mm, the amplitude of SEEG spikes would drop to 40%. This drop-off suggests that an electrode contact slightly farther away from the source may produce false-negative results. Therefore, a tight MEG cluster for MEG provides an essential

Fig. 5. Example case where the SEEG contacts involved had excellent sublobar concordance with a tight MEG cluster. The patient became seizure-free after resection of the co-identified cortical region by MEG and SEEG. *Blue spheres*, all implanted SEEG electrodes. *Red spheres*, ictal onset on SEEG. *Yellow spheres*, MEG dipole locations. A, anterior; P, posterior.

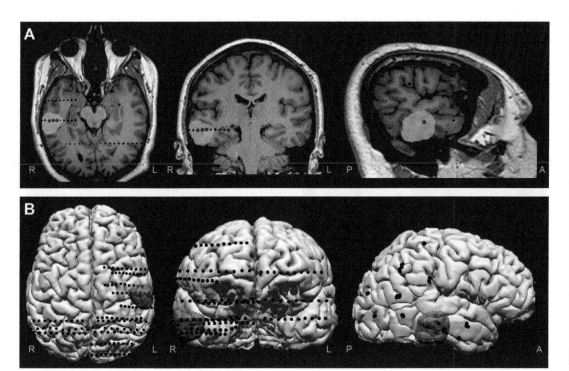

Fig. 6. Illustration of using the multimodal image integration platform for planning resection. The proposed resection area was interactively drawn on the MRI (coronal, axial, and sagittal views, *green region* in *A*), and can also be shown in 3D view together with the cortical surface (*orange region* in *B*). *Blue spheres* indicate all the implanted SEEG electrodes. A, anterior; L, left; P, posterior; R, right.

target for prospective designing of SEEG implantation. This is further supported by a recent study by Murakami and colleagues,[9] showing that patients had a significantly higher chance of being seizure-free when SEEG completely sampled the areas identified by MEG as compared with those with incomplete or no sampling of MEG results.

Using Magnetoencephalography to "Fill in the Gap" When Intracranial Electroencephalogram Has Limited Sampling

When the coverage of invasive EEG was inadequate, MEG integrated within a multimodal framework is used to remedy the situation by providing a synoptic view of whole-brain activities and "filling in the gaps" of invasive electrodes.[10] This is illustrated in **Fig. 7** with a patient who underwent presurgical evaluation with ICEEG and MEG. ICEEG showed a stable spike focus in the perirolandic region interictally, and ictal activities involved the same region, which would have been a difficult location for surgical resection. However, a consistent pattern of propagation was revealed by MEG sequential dipole analysis, showing interictal activity starting from the deep left parietal operculum/posterior insula and propagating to the primary and supplementary sensorimotor areas. This

example illustrates the situation where ICEEG data interpreted alone might bring misleading results because of epileptic activities emanating from deep structures propagating to cortical surface. Interpreting ICEEG results together with MEG may shed light on propagating activities on a millisecond by millisecond time resolution to "fill in the gaps" where there are no electrodes implanted.

Extraoperative and Intraoperative Use of Magnetoencephalography to Inform Resection Plan

Many previous studies have demonstrated that MEG can offer unique, nonredundant information to help identify implantation sites, when other noninvasive modalities' results are not illuminating.[9,11–14] Studies have also demonstrated that a single tight MEG cluster is a positive indicator of good seizure outcome, whereas patients with a loose MEG cluster or multiple clusters have less favorable outcomes.[9,13,15,16] A consensus from these studies is that a single tight cluster indicates a restricted epileptogenic generator, whereas a loose cluster or multiple clusters are suggestive of a more extensive epileptogenic region. Therefore, the location revealed by a

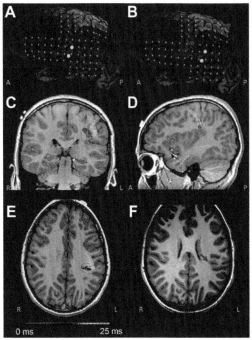

Fig. 7. Example of a patient with difficult-to-control seizures associated with a subtle focal cortical dysplasia residing within the deeper left parietal operculum and posterior insula, highlighting the potential benefits of dynamic analysis of interictal MEG propagation in the appropriate clinical context. (*A, B*) ICEEG reconstructed on top of a coregistered maximum intensity projection (MIP) image of the patient's MRI. *Green solid circles*, grid ICEEG electrodes; *cyan solid circles*, depth ICEEG electrodes targeting deeper structures; *red open circles*, interictally involved electrodes; *red solid circles*, ictally involved electrodes (involved depth electrode contacts not shown). (*C–E*) Results of MEG sequential dipole analysis of one interictal spike showing the trajectory of its propagation. This pattern was consistent across interictal spikes, starting from the left parietotemporal region and quickly propagating to the primary and supplementary motor cortex. Dipoles are sequentially fitted every 1 ms over 25 ms scale, and are shown in a color-coded time trajectory. Dipole positions are superimposed with the patient's MRI. (*F*) Prompted by the MEG findings, 3-T MRI with surface coil was performed, which confirmed a subtle dysplastic lesion at the onset location of the MEG interictal spike propagation (*red arrow*). Focal resection of this subtle lesion led to sustained seizure freedom in this patient. A, anterior; L, left; P, posterior; R, right.

conclusively positive tight MEG cluster should be targeted when designing the location and extent of the resection/ablation. This process could be done extraoperatively during the presurgical evaluation process, as illustrated in **Fig. 5**, and imported intraoperatively, as reported by a recent

study by Sommer and colleagues[17] including 28 patients with drug-resistant frontal lobe epilepsy who underwent resective surgery with intraoperative MEG guidance. The study examined separately patients with or without intraoperative MRI to navigate MEG foci during surgery, revealing a substantial difference in seizure outcomes (68% vs 50% seizure control rate). The integration of MEG with newer imaging techniques, such as MRI postprocessing, can also yield useful results for localization. In a recent study by Kasper and colleagues,[18] integration of MEG and MRI postprocessing demonstrated close spatial relationship between MEG source and type II focal cortical dysplasia (FCD) lesion with a circumscribed source localization in most patients; when the suspected epileptogenic zone identified by the combined MEG-MRI approach was completely resected, seizure-free rate was more than 80% after 3 years' follow-up. To echo this MEG-MRI approach, **Fig. 8** is an illustrative case where ICEEG data was overlaid with 2D MRI and 3D cortical surface rendering to reveal the proximity of a tight MEG cluster to a subtle depth of sulcus FCD lesion, which eventually led to a successful focal resection sparing language functions.

Magnetoencephalography-Guided Rereview of MRI

Results from MEG evaluation can also be used to guide rereview of the structural MRI. Not infrequently, such rereview can change the MRI study from negative to positive, when subtle structural changes are brought out by concordant electrophysiologic activities shown by the MEG. Moore and colleagues[20] reported 20 patients with neocortical epilepsy who were evaluated with MEG and MRI at 1.5-T; eight patients were initially determined as MRI negative. When retrospectively re-evaluated with the MEG information on MRI, four of the eight patients (50%) revealed a subtle transmantle sign on MRI. This is also illustrated in the previous example in **Fig. 7**. The benefit of MEG-guided MRI rereview also applies to ultrahigh-field MRI. In a recent study by Colon and colleagues,[21] 19 patients with focal epilepsy were scanned by a 7-T epilepsy protocol. Previously, there were no structural abnormalities on 3-T MRI in all 19 patients. The 7-T MRI by itself detected previously unseen structural abnormalities in 3 of the 19 patients; furthermore, with MEG guidance, 7-T MRI showed plausibly epileptogenic lesions in three more patients that were negative on 7-T/3-T MRI initially. It is important to note the implication of a new MRI lesion for

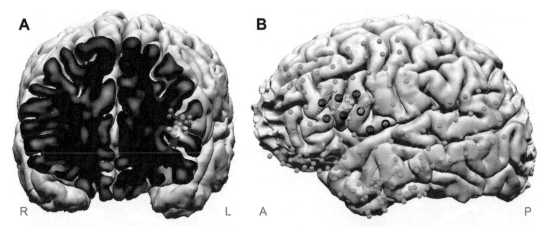

Fig. 8. Example of a patient in whom multimodal image integration revealed the proximity of a tight MEG cluster to a subtle depth-of-sulcus lesion. (*A*) Gray-white junction *z* score file from MRI postprocessing,[19] fused with the 3D cortical surface generated by Freesurfer. The high *z* score region on the gray-white junction file reveals a subtle depth-of-sulcus FCD (shown by the arrow) that was overlooked before. *Yellow spheres* indicate the location of a tight interictal MEG dipole cluster that overlapped with the FCD location. (*B*) ICEEG ictal findings (performed using subdural grids and depth electrodes), which were highly concordant with the lesion location. *Spheres* indicate the location of all implanted electrode contacts; *green*, all electrodes; *red*, ictal onset; *blue/magenta*, contacts where electrical stimulation showed slow/stop reading indicating the location of speech area. This patient underwent resective surgery, which completely included the depth-of-sulcus FCD lesion/MEG cluster. Histopathology revealed FCD type IIB. The patient was seizure-free for 1 year at the most recent follow-up with no language deficits. A, anterior; L, left; P, posterior; R, right.

the presurgical evaluation process, because MRI–positive patients were reported to be twice as likely to become seizure-free as MRI–negative patients.[22] To solidify the confidence of the subtle abnormality based on MEG-guided rereview of the MRI, it is often necessary to review the MEG-indicated area in multiple MRI sequences (T1-, T2-, or T2*-weighted), and accurate coregistration of the MEG results and MRI sequences is essential for the process. When adopted under the multimodal image integration framework, this comparison is made fairly straightforward.

Using Magnetoencephalography to Inform Evaluation of Surgical Failures

When faced with a patient with previously failed surgery for evaluation of possible reoperation, multimodal integration can often generate additional information. All the data collected from the previous evaluation (if available) and the current evaluation should be put together to understand the relevance of the multiple modalities to postulate the reasons for failure, and to inform the generation of electroclinical hypotheses for the current evaluation. Integrating the postoperative MRI and evaluating the extent of surgical cavity may shed light on what might have been missing (eg, Did the previous invasive evaluation not have adequate coverage? Was the ictal onset zone

only partially resected?) Once these factors are identified, consideration of further steps for reoperation may be more straightforward. El Tahry and colleagues[23] performed a retrospective study that included a consecutive cohort of 46 patients who failed prior resective epilepsy surgery, underwent re-evaluation including MEG and ictal SPECT, and had another surgery after the re-evaluation. The study showed that resection of the MEG localization was positively associated with a favorable outcome, whereas resection of the ictal SPECT localization was positively associated with a favorable outcome only in the early injection subgroup. **Fig. 9** illustrates one patient whose MEG cluster location guided the resection, which was completely removed and the patient became seizure-free.

FUTURE DIRECTIONS

In most prior studies, the simple single equivalent current dipole model was used for localization of MEG, which is consistent with the accepted practice in the clinical MEG community.[5] As Tenney and colleagues[24] reported, the use of multiple types of source estimation methods in addition to SECD modeling, such as dipole scanning, beamforming, or current density reconstruction, may optimize the strengths and limit the weaknesses of each individual algorithm. Integration

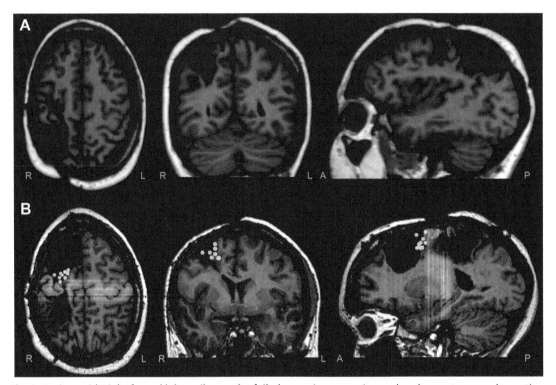

Fig. 9. Patient with right frontal lobe epilepsy who failed a previous resection and underwent a second resection. The patient's ictal MEG showed a tight cluster, whereas interictal MEG was negative. The previous resection was multilobar involving right perirolandic and parietal areas. The MEG focus was included in the second resection, and the patient became seizure-free. Surgical pathology showed FCD type I. (*A*) Resection from the first surgery, which did not render the patient seizure-free. (*B*) Right frontal lobe resection from the second surgery, which did render the patient seizure-free. *Yellow spheres* indicate the location of MEG dipoles, which were included in the second surgery. A, anterior; L, left; P, posterior; R, right.

of localization results from these methods into the multimodal framework for interictal and ictal MEG localization may further inform understanding of the epileptic network.

Furthermore, the utility of multimodal image integration should not merely stop at displaying all the presurgical evaluation data. As a next step, using seizure outcome data and postoperative MRI from previous surgical cases, it is conceivable that quantitative approaches could be developed to suggest an "optimal plan" for implantation schemes and resection planning. Because of the large amount of multimodal data associated with this process, machine learning approaches could be leveraged for improved computational scalability.

SUMMARY

This article emphasizes the importance of adopting a 3D multimodal image integration approach in epilepsy presurgical evaluation. The success of SEEG explorations is enhanced, when integrating a preoperative MEG to implantation

planning. Assessing concordance between MEG and other tests can provide essential and complimentary information for generating surgical hypothesis, electrode trajectory planning, interpreting ICEEG data, designing the final resection, and addressing surgical failures. It is our hope that multimodal image integration including MEG plays a more frequent role in epilepsy presurgical evaluation.

DISCLOSURE

None.

REFERENCES

1. Engel J Jr, Wiebe S, French J, et al. Practice parameter: temporal lobe and localized neocortical resections for epilepsy: report of the Quality Standards Subcommittee of the American Academy of Neurology, in association with the American Epilepsy Society and the American Association of Neurology. Neurology 2003;60(4): 538–47.

2. Choi H, Sell RL, Lenert L, et al. Epilepsy surgery for pharmacoresistant temporal lobe epilepsy: a decision analysis. JAMA 2008; 300(21):2497–505.

3. Fauser S. Factors influencing surgical outcome in patients with focal cortical dysplasia. J Neurol Neurosurg Psychiatry 2008;79:103–5.

4. O'Brien TJ, So EL, Mullan BP, et al. Subtraction ictal SPECT co-registered to MRI improves clinical usefulness of SPECT in localizing the surgical seizure focus. Neurology 1998;50(2):445–54.

5. Bagic AI, Knowlton RC, Rose DF, et al. American Clinical Magnetoencephalography Society Clinical Practice Guideline 1: Recording and Analysis of Spontaneous Cerebral Activity. J Clin Neurophysiol 2011;28(4):348–54.

6. LaViolette Peter S, Rand Scott D, Ellingson Benjamin M, et al. 3D visualization of subdural electrode shift as measured at craniotomy reopening. Epilepsy Res 2011;94(1–2):102–9.

7. Nowell M, Rodionov R, Zombori G, et al. Utility of 3D multimodality imaging in the implantation of intracranial electrodes in epilepsy. Epilepsia 2015. https://doi.org/10.1111/epi.12924.

8. Kakisaka Y, Kubota Y, Wang ZI, et al. Use of simultaneous depth and MEG recording may provide complementary information regarding the epileptogenic region. Epileptic Disord 2012;14(3):298–303.

9. Murakami H, Wang ZI, Marashly A, et al. Correlating magnetoencephalography to stereoelectroencephalography in patients undergoing epilepsy surgery. Brain 2016;139:2935–47.

10. Wang ZI, Jin K, Kakisaka Y, et al. Imag(in)ing seizure propagation: MEG-guided interpretation of epileptic activity from a deep source. Hum Brain Mapp 2012; 33(12):2797–801.

11. Mamelak AN, Lopez N, Akhtari M, et al. Magnetoencephalography-directed surgery in patients with neocortical epilepsy. J Neurosurg 2002;97(97): 865–73.

12. Sutherling W, Mamelak AN, Thyerlei D, et al. Influence of magnetic source imaging for planning intracranial EEG in epilepsy. Neurology 2008;71(13): 990–6.

13. Knowlton Robert C, Razdan Shantanu N, Limdi N, et al. Effect of epilepsy magnetic source imaging on intracranial electrode placement. Ann Neurol 2009;65(6):716–23.

14. Agirre-Arrizubieta Z, Thai Ngoc J, Valentin A, et al. The value of magnetoencephalography to guide electrode implantation in epilepsy. Brain Topogr 2014;27(1):197–207.

15. Oishi M, Kameyama S, Masuda H, et al. Single and multiple clusters of magnetoencephalographic dipoles in neocortical epilepsy: significance in characterizing the epileptogenic zone. Epilepsia 2006; 47(2):355–64.

16. Almubarak S, Alexopoulos A, Von-Podewils F, et al. The correlation of magnetoencephalography to intracranial EEG in localizing the epileptogenic zone: a study of the surgical resection outcome. Epilepsy Res 2014;108(9):1581–90.

17. Sommer B, Roessler K, Rampp S, et al. Magnetoencephalography-guided surgery in frontal lobe epilepsy using neuronavigation and intraoperative MR imaging. Epilepsy Res 2016;126:26–36.

18. Kasper BS, Rössler K, Hamer Hajo M, et al. Coregistrating magnetic source and magnetic resonance imaging for epilepsy surgery in focal cortical dysplasia. Neuroimage Clin 2018;19:487–96.

19. Wang ZI, Jones SE, Jaisani Z, et al. Voxel-based morphometric magnetic resonance imaging (MRI) postprocessing in MRI-negative epilepsies. Ann Neurol 2015;77(6):1060–75.

20. Moore KR, Funke ME, Constantino T, et al. Magnetoencephalographically directed review of high-spatial-resolution surface-coil MR images improves lesion detection in patients with extratemporal epilepsy. Radiology 2002;225(3):880–7.

21. Colon AJ, Osch MJPV, Buijs M, et al. MEG-guided analysis of 7T-MRI in patients with epilepsy. Seizure 2018;60:29–38.

22. Tellez-Zenteno JF, Hernandez Ronquillo L, Moien-Afshari F, et al. Surgical outcomes in lesional and non-lesional epilepsy: a systematic review and meta-analysis. Epilepsy Res 2010;89(2–3):310–8.

23. El Tahry R, Wang ZI, Thandar A, et al. Magnetoencephalography and ictal SPECT in patients with failed epilepsy surgery. Clin Neurophysiol 2018; 129(8):1651–7.

24. Tenney JR, Fujiwara H, Horn Paul S, et al. Comparison of magnetic source estimation to intracranial EEG, resection area, and seizure outcome. Epilepsia 2014;55(11):1854–63.